DEDICATION

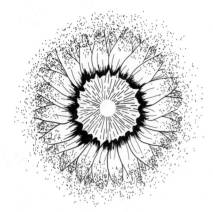

This book is dedicated with love to Lesley Tippitt, whose generosity, clarity, and devotion to the Bragg Legacy— and to the health and happiness of women worldwide— delivered this book into your hands.

ACKNOWLEDGEMENTS

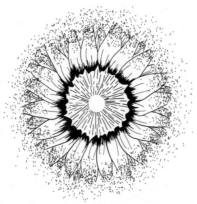

First, I would like to thank *the one and only* Patricia Bragg for dedicating her life to the message that every person deserves to be as healthy and happy as possible. Because of her tenacity, wit, and wisdom, I am alive and kicking—as are millions of others. Patricia, I am deeply honored to share your secrets for ageless beauty with the world.

To Lesley Tippitt, one of the smartest and kindest women on the planet. Thank you for inviting me into the circle, giving me the opportunity of a lifetime and a friendship I cherish. I promise you that next year we'll work less, as I don't think it's possible to work more. Here's to self-care and a dozen facials.

To Jen Bolton, your eye for detail and willingness to persevere is astounding and acknowledged. To Fallon McConville. for the magnificent sunflower image which captured the wildness of Revolutionary Beauty.

To Jane Lamp, for her enthusiastic support, ready smile, and facility with all things technical. To Michelle Ratliff, for your heartfelt assistance with social media.

To the clients who have trusted me with your healing journey, and dug deep to reclaim your birthright of health and vitality—you taught me everything I know. I love you all.

To Dr. Julia T. Hunter, MD; Dr. Leigh Connealy, MD; Dr. Rey Alcerro, DC; Dr. Robert Cass, ND; Dr. Dale Migliaccio, DC; Dr. Darin Bunch, OMD; Dr. Julie Taguchi, MD; Dr. Robert Weiser, DDS; Dr. Michael Galitzer, MD; Linda Turner; Torrey Trover; Madelyn Reusser; and Brenda Ogeslby—the medical doctors, naturopaths, homeopaths, chiropractors, lymphatic drainage therapists, and acupuncturists I call "my team." Thank you for opening your hearts and minds to my work and clients.

To Julia Molino, for your elegant and exquisite sense of organization, your delicate fine-tuning and superb editing skills—and for seeing the possibilities in this project when it was but a twinkle in Spirit's eye.

To Deborah S. Nelson, without whom my books would not see the light of day! Here we are again, and I'm so thankful—for your gorgeous cover design, interior graphics, editing, website support—what can't you do? Thank you also to Sara Winner, for the long hours.

To Kenny, for modeling creativity at its best—openhearted, with a leap of faith. A deep bow for walking with me through the rocky landscape of my *beauty-wound* and inspiring me to heal—though it took decades. Thank you for writing the foreword to this book, and for teaching us all that anything is possible.

To Luke, your sensitivity, integrity, and intelligence match the radiance of your heart. I am honored to partner with you; to be your student as you share your spirit, skills, instincts—and your humor. There is no end to the tapestry with which you will weave your healing gifts.

To Hana, the Revolutionary Beauty who challenged me from the day you were born to find my voice, be authentic, and stay in the ring—as you do. Your fierce tenderness, wonderful laugh, and capacity to love surges through your music and soul like lightning. Your songwriting is a gift. I am in awe, daily.

To the best sister in the world—and best aunt—Susan Cooper Taublieb. While the world knows you as the cocreator of The Manadoob Program for Social and Emotional Learning, and a spectacular director and producer, I am blessed that you are my brilliant, savvy, and fun best friend who is stuck with me because we're related!

To my nephews, Zev, Ari, and Noah, for gently inviting your mom and me to become much better people! We will keep at it. I am humbled by your work ethic, and your devotion to each other and our family.

To Paul Taublieb, for always being in our corner when we need you. Thank you for taking such good care of my sister and those gorgeous boys.

To Cointa, Miguel, and Lino Trujillo Reveles, our other family. I cannot imagine life without the love, adventures, and connection we share.

To the dear friends who love me in all my seasons: Clovis and Grady, Peter Pomeranze, Adela Barcia, Angelique Millette, Samantha Friedland, Amy Wilson, Judith Smith, Diane Murphy, Lisa Proctor Hawkins, Crystal Cass, Georgia Schockley, Bill Culman, Marilyn Miller, and Chuck Blitz.

Finally, with all my love and gratitude, to my husband, Paul Turner, the ground beneath my feet. Your integrity, generosity, and character are unparalleled. I love you. Thank you for making me feel safe and loved, every single day, for ten years. Thank you for sharing me with my life's work, never complaining, except to remind me to eat, sleep, and breathe. This book could not have been written without your unconditional support and unwavering belief in me.

—Julia Loggins

FOREWORD

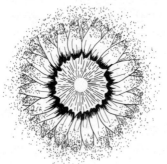

By Kenny Loggins

When I first heard that Julia was writing a book on beauty, I had to chuckle to myself ...

"Do you mean the Julia I know? I don't know anyone more conflicted about her beauty than she. How could she write a credible book of advice about that?" And, then I realized, "Of course! That is **so** Julia! Who better to understand the internal struggle between one's authenticity and one's outward presentation? She's been working on that all her life. She **must** be an authority by now."

Ok ... So it's 1991 ... I recall taking her shopping for clothes when we were first together. She's trying on clothes, looking at herself modeling a designer dress, staring glassy-eyed into the full-length mirror, and suddenly she starts crying. Weeping! I had no clue why. To me, in that moment she was simply a pretty girl in the wrong dress. I didn't understand it then, but I would eventually learn that she just couldn't be objective when it came to assessing her look. Her inner critic was so angry, so loud, she couldn't hear me tell her how beautiful she actually was. "This looks good on me," just wasn't in her vocabulary.

Once, when we were doing an interview for *Home and Garden TV* showing off our new home, the interviewer inquired, "It's so unusual for the husband to be so involved with the interiors. Usually, the husband does the landscaping and the wife does the interior decorating."

To which I replied, "Oh, it's that way here. Julia is very much in charge of the interior—rather, she is in charge of the *spiritual interior* of our home—which is everything you don't see."

I saw early in our love affair that Julia was actually a stunning beauty in disguise. When she would put it together, get really dressed up, what we called "clean up," she could be jaw-dropping. Her face was a showstopper, with a sunny California style and a million dollar smile. Her brief modeling career even took her to Japan, where she did a stint on camera as a weather girl. But her war with herself never let up, and it always seemed like the cleaned up, Prada version of Julia was too uncomfortable as if she wore in an inauthentic disguise.

No matter how much positive feedback she got for her looks, what Julia now refers to as her beauty-wound could not be healed from the outside in. As time went by, I assumed my love would help that heal, but it wasn't to be. She had to go in to get out. This riddle would only be solved as an inside job.

Unbeknownst to me, my role back then was to be her *change agent*, to take her into the belly of the beast, the *red carpets* of my life that would be so incredibly challenging for her. Where I thought I was taking her on a fun, wild ride into *the world*, instead my life would take her into her pain, to her edge, and ultimately to her *Self*.

So, my role now is to be the witness to the struggle her spirit had with beauty itself. The Julia I knew was always a spiritual warrior, the kind of woman who would keep looking inward for the answers no matter the cost.

I now realize this book was inevitable because it was inevitable that her beauty demons would eventually succumb to her dogged emotional scrutiny. Her struggle is exactly what brings credibility to this book. It's the inner journey that brings peace, and it's the inner peace that creates beauty.

So, this is the culmination of a lifetime of following the bread crumbs, the clues that would eventually lead her home. If you can relate to her struggle—if you still feel like a stranger in a strange land—you just might find your own keys *out of hell* here.

As a songwriter all my life, I learned early on that if I could tell my story as vulnerably and honestly as possible, people would see their own story in that song. The personal is the universal.

This is Julia's song.

Feel free to dance.

—Kenny Loggins
Singer and Songwriter

PREFACE

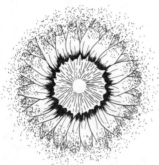

By Julia Loggins

Iconic health crusader, organic gardening pioneer, and co-founder of the first American natural foods product company, Patricia Bragg, radiantly ageless, is reinventing her life.

This health forerunner, world-renowned speaker, and media powerhouse is dedicating the next decade to her message that everyone deserves radiant health and happiness. She believes each of us has the ability to transform our physical health, energy, attitude, and habits to live an extraordinary life—a life free of limitation and pain. Her dream for you is to inspire a life full of possibility, where beauty and age are redefined, with opportunity ahead—regardless of age—and with nothing to prove.

The time has come to eliminate the rhetoric that narrowly defines beauty as an unachievable ideal. When we shed layers of conditioning that say self-worth evaporates after 40, we realize our true power and ability to experience pleasure. That potent truth liberates us from the lie and opens us to fresh, new possibilities.

Patricia Bragg is revolutionizing not only what we "eat, breathe, think, say, and do," but shows us how to glide into the last third of our lives in vibrant health, and embrace who we are. She is passionate about leading women to be "the captains of their own ship," and sometimes a pirate—free from needing permission, validation, or acceptance.

She believes in women practicing radical truth—to smile when we look in the mirror. How do we do this? We purify our precious bodies, prioritize mental health, soothe burn-out with breath work and choose fasting and natural food over fad diets. When we embrace creativity over condition-ing and sensuality over service, we release the lines on our faces and the angst in our souls—and we change the world!

A call to arms—linked arms—starts with women unapolo-getically healing ourselves and every life force on the planet. This starts with the revolutionary willingness to stop com-paring the way we look to other women. Instead, we glow with the perfection of our imperfect natures. Rather than starving ourselves, we delight in healthy food and bodies. True beauty is about joy, not suffering. Beauty is built, as is vitality, from the inside out. Anyone can do it.

We will show you how, step by step.

Women have been conditioned since birth to feel small. This manifests in eating disorders, holding back words, and fear of taking up space. When we walk shyly instead of prancing with our heads held high, we diminish authenticity. A piece of our soul dies—and nothing ages us more.

Patricia Bragg's sparkling smile fills the room. Through an unshakable confidence in the simple laws of Mother Nature, she trusts her authority to speak, rather than shrink. From knowing her, that confidence and authority are contagious! You will feel it pour over you on these pages, like fairy dust.

We have the right to stand for what we know to be true. Often, self-sabotaging toxins held in our bodies and brains disable our perfectly tuned inner GPS. Once we detoxify and reset our inner GPS, we are guided toward choices such as writing in a journal over wolfing down a pint of ice cream. This book gives you tools to win that wrestling match with cravings and hands you the keys out of hell.

Inner authority is beauty *and* power. When we don't feel beautiful, we are not inhabiting the range of our power, within ourselves or the world. And, as I discovered as a young woman, rebelling from society's idea of beauty doesn't heal the beauty-wound. We must heal from the inside. When beauty doesn't exist merely as a projection from the world, we own it. And instead of diminishing, true beauty grows. You become ageless.

That is when the magic begins. That's what this book is about.

Patricia Bragg's genuine beauty, power, and radiance have transformed and motivated women of all ages. And with Patricia's blessing, my mission is to revolutionize the culture of beauty, through the time-tested Bragg Healthy Lifestyle.

—Julia Loggins

TABLE OF CONTENTS

INTRODUCTION

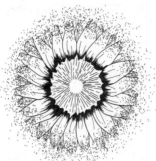

What is Beauty?
MEET PATRICIA

The first time I met Patricia Bragg in the flesh, her reputation as *The Queen of Natural Living* preceded her. But what struck me was her sparkling energy. I could feel her 50 yards away. Her eyes shined, her smile beamed, and her skin was crystal clear and nearly wrinkle-free. Her jaw was taut and firm as if she was 30-something. And yet, she must have been at least … what? Ageless! Nothing sagged, and I mean, nothing. Although she's only 4' 10" (4' 11" in pink cowboy boots), she is, as she says with a twinkle, "a giant of a woman, because my message is a giant one."

Have you ever looked at pictures of family members in their youth, and couldn't recognize them? Did you ever go to a high school reunion and gasp upon seeing an old friend, who barely resembled their graduation picture?

Not Patricia Bragg. In her nineties, she is as magnetic as in the days when she circled the globe with Paul Bragg. This dynamic duo inspired three generations of health food enthusiasts and cajoled business owners to start this newfangled invention called a health food store.

Patricia is devoted to the ministry of health and happiness—not fashion trends. Yet, she adores playing with clothes, shoes, hats, and sparkling jewelry. Her technicolor rainbow style—bright pink, mango, lavender, rose, and gold—shouts unapologetically, "Here I am!" *The Queen's* self-confidence emanates from her evangelical mission of wellness for all and a fearless protection of a planet. Though these were radical concepts in the 1950s, she never considered herself a revolutionary. Still, the battle cry, "Don't panic, it's organic," was a bold challenge to the conventional chemical farming methods she fought her entire life. Her radiance, power, and resilience springs from her passion and love for Mother Earth. When you meet Patricia Bragg, you cannot look away. Her energy emits a force field.

Beauty is an Inside Job

The University College in London's Wellcome Laboratory of Neurobiology published a report showing that beauty exists as an abstract concept within the brain. Cultural conditioning teaches us that certain body types and facial features are deemed more attractive than others. In his book, *Deviate: The Science of Seeing Differently*, neuroscientist Beau Lotto explains that the mind does not see reality. The mind creates stories based on biological and physiological assumptions. These assumptions can be either inherited, experienced, or influenced by cultural conditioning.

He says when we change our actions and how we feel about ourselves, we literally alter the way the world sees us.

Research proves that the brain perceives inner sparkle and self-assurance as authentic beauty and desirability. Human beings are designed to be irresistibly attracted to both. We're like fireflies drawn to the light on a moonless August eve—we can't stay away from beauty. So, how do we unwind from society's definition of beauty and create our own?

And that takes me to Grace.

I will never forget Grace—one of the most popular girls in high school. Grace wasn't a cheerleader or prom queen. I recall hearing our algebra teacher describe her as "handsome," not exactly a compliment in the era of Playboy Bunnies and Twiggy. A head taller than most of the boys and like an Olympic swimmer with broad shoulders, Grace had long, strong arms and muscular legs. You felt her enter the room. Everyone looked her way, smiled, and took a deep breath. She carried herself with elegance, even when her skin was *having a bad day*. Every boy wanted to date her, and every girl wanted to be her friend. I puzzled over that. Grace wasn't skinny, blonde, or giggly. She wasn't trying to get attention. She seemed so comfortable in her own skin. *How did she become her?* I wondered. *How can I become my version of Grace?*

My sense is that a parent or grandparent—someone close—adored her. Or, maybe they were too busy keeping a roof over their heads to mess with her mojo. One thing is certain: Grace's beauty sprung from the inside and radiated like the aurora borealis. Her confidence had nothing to do with the symmetry of her features, breast size, or hip quotient. Unmistakably hers, she was not competing or comparing. Her dignity worked like a hypnotic charm, and we were all crazy about her.

In May of our senior year, Harvard offered Grace a scholarship. I thought, "She's beautiful **and** smart!" I was happy for her—you couldn't hate Grace—but it was almost too much. How did she do it? The truth is, her brain wasn't scrambled trying to figure how to be seen or stay invisible; how to maneuver a date for Saturday night; or what to wear to look attractive. The foundation of desirability is self-acceptance; a healthy, balanced sense of entitlement; and the right to go after our dreams. The right to be beautiful. The right to be powerful. The right to be ageless.

How do mere mortals achieve this? If we have been bumped and bruised by life, as most have, this level of self-love may seem a lofty goal. Where do we even start?

We start by healing burnout, brain fog, chronic pain, and fatigue. These are the enemies that steal joy, wrinkle skin, and squash creativity. What is the real *fountain of youth?* Energy—boundless, unstoppable energy and optimism, the willingness to take risks and try new things.

That's the power and zest I felt beaming from Patricia Bragg when I first met her, and what many lose with age. The goal of this book is to rekindle the faith that *anything is possible, at any age.* As Kelly LeBrock says, the word "revolution" means to create a sharp change, and that is exactly the recipe for Revolutionary Beauty.

Revolutionary Beauty is timeless, sourced from within. The conventional beauty model is one defined by others and designed to be discarded. Fueled by profit and greed, soul and spirit are given little consideration. We need to create and embody ageless renewable energy. Therefore, we focus on that which values life, resources, and natural authenticity for ourselves and the planet.

That is exactly what "The CARE Plan" does: **C**reates **A**geless **R**enewable **E**nergy to benefit all. This seven-step program is based on the time-tested Bragg Healthy Lifestyle, and the dynamic practices that I have taught for the last 40 years, proven to heal and regenerate. "The CARE Plan" was created to inspire freedom and flow and to ignite your Vital Force. Everything you need to heal resides within you.

We will teach you how to release stress and trauma—toxins as destructive as any chemical. You will purify, fuel, and move your body to create more energy than you've ever experienced. The skin is the largest organ of your body, and even the most expensive and potent facial creams penetrate only the two top layers. Patricia's luminescence emanates from the vitality of her organs, and the rituals we'll share. These include Mother Nature's secrets for building collagen and reducing lines. Revolutionary Beauty is built step by step and when you complete these steps, you'll own your own brand of beauty.

You will meet Revolutionary Beauties who will inspire and ignite you to make your dreams come true. This means prioritizing creativity and reinventing—instead of retiring. Some of the Revolutionary Beauties mentioned in this book began their first businesses in their sixties! Revolutionary Beauty comes from finding your purpose and living your joy. We need you. The planet needs you. And your spirit needs **you**. *This is the heroine's journey.*

Here's to you, Revolutionary Beauty! Clean Deep. Glow Bright. Change the world!

—Julia Loggins

CHAPTER 1

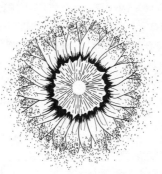

JULIA'S STORY

*"What is the point, if even
beautiful women are wounded, too?"*

—Julia Loggins, Digestive Health Expert and Author

The subject of women's beauty is ancient and complex and has perplexed me relentlessly, like a compelling riddle to be solved. Then, I met a woman who embodied beauty as effortlessly as the moon illuminates the sky. Confident and joyful, in pink boots and a cowboy hat, she built an empire and changed the world. Patricia's contagious passion inspired me to capture what magic drove this dynamo to live outside the cultural conditioning with which I had fought and rebelled against. What fairy dust fueled her desire to teach millions to do the same? I was compelled to discover her secrets.

My foray into the world of beauty began with unlikely circumstances. To heal a jagged relationship with my body, my therapist suggested that I shoot a modeling portfolio. Through a friend, these images landed on an agent's desk at Wilhemina, one of the largest modeling agencies in the world. To my surprise, they immediately signed me.

Since I spent my first twenty years frequently hospitalized with life-threatening asthma, scoliosis, and rheumatoid arthritis—bald and eyebrowless from experimental drug therapies—this was not a predictable scenario. In fact, doctors told my parents I wouldn't live to be 17. However, a medical doctor influenced by natural health trailblazer Paul Bragg, and his exuberant daughter, Patricia, wrote an unusual *prescription*. This prescription called for an all-organic diet that eliminated sugar, wheat, dairy, processed foods, and chemicals—and, slowly, all my pharmaceutical medications. This protocol and believing healing was possible, saved my life.

Resurrected, my focus turned to learn everything about how to rebuild my health. However, fate had a detour in store. As a wild child living in Venice, California, I met and married a therapist. David was a survivor of Auschwitz, 25 years my senior, and a protégé of Bob Hoffman of the Hoffman Institute. The Institute is a personal growth retreat founded in the 1960s to help people heal from trauma. David gave me two assignments.

The first was to get in touch with the unconscious rage he believed was crippling my body. I didn't know I had rage. *Me, angry?* I was grateful to be alive. I'd been dancing on my grave all my life—dancing fast and furious. When everyone around me was terrified of my imminent demise, I was relentlessly sunny and positive. Feeling fear, or any uncomfortable feeling, was an inconvenient luxury.

David challenged me to dip below the surface to find my voice—the "**No!**" I had never uttered. "No!" to the medicines that caused side effects, "No!' to countless needle punctures, and "No!" to being told I was crazy. A colleague of his, a progressive psychiatrist, lent me her soundproofed, padded bright red office in Brentwood. Each night I writhed and pounded pillows. This was my opportunity to tell a few people things I could never say. I ended each session with a prayer of compassion for myself, and for them.

Eighteen months later, I was an inch and a half taller. My scoliosis had healed, and my spine was straight.

The second assignment David gave me was intended as a lighthearted invitation. He wanted me to experiment with feeling beautiful and sexy, words that felt like distant descriptions of someone else. He wanted me to meet and mingle with the someone elses who owned the *title of Beautiful*, and to experience their world.

As someone who spent her childhood breathing through tubes rather than playing with makeup, no one was more surprised than I that the assigned photo shoot launched a modeling career. My lack of digestive health and inability to absorb nutrients assured me that my 5'5" frame barely held 105 pounds with my boots on. This made me, in the words of my agent, "perfect." At 23, I had never worn lipstick. My head was still partially bald. But there I was, cowboy hat in hand, headed off into the wild blue yonder of catwalks and bright lights. At that moment, the cowboy hat and my organic diet were about all I had in common with my hero, *The Queen of Natural Living*, Patricia Bragg.

I had much to learn, and Spirit was about to teach me.

Welcome to Hollywood.

Nervous and naive, I was catapulted into the industry. Compassionate stylists combed my hair over bald parts, and photographers made me laugh. I found myself in a world of women who had been told they were beautiful all their lives. They would teach me about beauty, I imagined. I would soak up their sureness. They would hand confidence to me like a tapestry, which I would drape around my shoulders to feel beautiful. And the oddest part of it all were these vessels of feminine symmetry who were to teach me how to feel desirable. Well, they were torturing themselves day and night with more self-trash-talk than pro wrestlers in the WWF.

I was gob-smacked. I, who had logged as many hours in the ICU as they had spent playing dress-up, held more self-esteem. And, believe me, I felt next to none. *How does that happen?* I wondered. *What is beauty, anyway? What is the point, if even beautiful women are wounded, too?*

What I discovered in my modeling career was that no woman in the western world escapes the conditioning that shapes what is considered beautiful. I also learned that rebelling is not freedom. If anything, rebellion intensifies this depth of conditioning and how we're each affected. Humans are hardwired to be attracted to beauty—it's in our DNA.

Yet, we can reframe what beauty means and become architects of its creation. We can own the keys to the temple. Like nature, in its purest form, female beauty is both grounded and luminous. When we are vibrantly healthy, blissfully happy, and authentically present, we shine. Just as the moon is awe-inspiring, so are we.

I didn't discover this on a runway. In fact, my beauty-wound went deeper underground. Just two years into my modeling career, my once again failing health demanded I do whatever was needed to heal my body, once and for all. The travel and inability to get healthy foods took a toll. Asthma and allergies reappeared with a vengeance. This required me to resume my 100 percent organic diet *and* add a detoxifying regimen of juicing to regenerate my organs. I drank gallons of wheatgrass juice to nourish my starving brain and surrendered to the relentless rules of regenerative health. In other words, I embraced life in Patricia Bragg's entire universe. By doing so, I completely recreated and renewed my body, in a way I never imagined I could.

By the next year, I was devoted to helping others heal. My modeling days were behind me, and so was wearing lipstick and owning more than three dresses. I was happier than I'd ever been, having found *my tribe* and my life's work.

David supported me to work only with "those who are fighting for their life as you fought for yours." We didn't have much, but life in the little studio above my office was good. As the song says, "We don't have money, even though I'm so in love with you honey ..."

With 35-year-old hormones raging, baby fever grabbed me by the throat and would not let go. David and I divorced—he didn't want children. I met and married the handsome guy who wrote that same love song, Kenny Loggins. Soon I was in front of a camera again, forced to face the beauty-wound, in love with a man who millions of other women wanted, too. Gorgeous women. Blond women. Tall women. And, let's not forget about women with certain body parts in sizes I did not possess.

At 35, I had experienced the satisfaction of a successful career in progressive health. I saw myself as doing serious work that seemed more important than the latest trend in *Vogue Magazine*. And, I had spent years addressing the traumas of my youth. The beauty-wound that I thought I was beyond terrified and infuriated me. I had no idea that just being a woman in America means there is nowhere to go and nowhere to hide. Society's definition of beauty is inside us—an invisible set of punishing rules that we use against ourselves. Deep inside me, I discovered one of the few toxins I had not yet flushed from my system—unworthiness. Kenny saw me as beautiful when all I saw was the bald, skinny, flat chested girl of my youth.

During this time, I learned how inextricably beauty and power are connected. Even though part of me was basking in the bliss of love, another part of me was sabotaging myself. I didn't undermine myself by stuffing my mouth with cookies, because sugar makes me violently ill. I shrunk, constantly comparing myself to lovely, younger women who—and they were always around—we would meet on the road. I felt unworthy of love and this new, extraordinary life.

Kenny was not immune to society's rules either. His career was the perfect arena for a wrestling match with the *beauty jones*—the elusive holy grail that entices men to be attracted to women of physical perfection. Although he never acted on them, the constant temptations loomed everywhere. I always felt I had to compete, and the pressure drove me crazy. Like many men, Kenny didn't grow up seeing himself as the smart, handsome guy he was. When he felt confused or fearful—or was taking a leap of faith into new territory—in his mind, he became the skinny, bucktoothed 17-year-old Kenny who couldn't land a date. And now he was the Crown Prince of Pop. He loved me. Yet, his conditioning as an American male was to compare me to what else was available.

How could he not? How many men have soaked in the unique experience of being wanted, adored, and fantasized about by millions of women?

Under this microscope, the fiery spotlight of fame, we each simmered in our insecurities. And yet, we knew we had a phenomenal opportunity to face a beast that his career did not create, but only revealed. That beast was all we were taught by well-meaning parents and society about beauty and self-worth. Many times, my fear was so intense that I wanted to run away. In fact, once I did. I climbed out the window of our bedroom while he was being interviewed by *Good Morning, America*, a story we tell in our book, *The Unimaginable Life*.

When we let ourselves open our hearts, we found compassion for ourselves and for each other. We learned there is no way out, but in. We did our best to become allies, rather than victims or perpetrators.

Through the process of writing *The Unimaginable Life*—and the twists and turns that came after—I learned something that changed my life. Because he was male and successful, I felt Kenny held all the power. Over time, I discovered that I, too, had power—and that it was within me all along.

When I became receptive to that power, everyone and everything around me changed.

To nurture and maintain a daily awareness of self-love and inner power takes time. Yet, transformation can occur in an instant—often birthed through crisis. When we're most lost—on our knees in pain—we shed the armor we believe protects us, and open ourselves to discoveries that change our lives forever. An agonizing third miscarriage led me to such a discovery: my inner power, the power of the mind— and its amazing connection to the body.

The day after this miscarriage, I read a magazine article about the work of a trailblazing therapist, Niravi Payne. She pioneered a new way to heal infertility through the release of negative beliefs and emotional blocks. Her program led to the birth of 5,000 precious babies.

I immediately called her. She answered with a thick New York accent, "Hello, Bubby, who is this?"

At that moment, I wasn't sure. I had just lost a baby on a flight between Miami and Los Angeles. I let her talk. We clicked. She asked what seemed like a thousand questions about my childhood, life, and health history. She was quiet for a moment. Then she delivered her diagnosis in a calm, stern voice: "Julia, you're holding so much stress in your body that your womb is a kettle of boiling acid, unable to sustain life—any life—even your own."

That took me by surprise! I had come so far. To think that a mountain was still in front of me was daunting. Yet, I didn't care about the climb. I wanted to be a mother.

Niravi and I had slightly different, though intersecting agendas. While I focused on birthing a baby, she focused on me birthing myself. She chose the field of fertility because she believed women longing to be mothers are the most motivated group of people alive. I checked all the boxes. Desperate. Dedicated. Determined.

Isn't that always when the miracles happen?

We began with phone sessions. The first thing that Niravi did was to send me a biofeedback card, a handy device that uses body heat to reveal stress through color codes. This was to measure just how hot that kettle of mine boiled. If one is *yogi level calm*, the card turns blue. Still tranquil, but with an active mind, green. Stressed—beginning to burn—red. Black—shut your mouth—make no decisions and breathe into a paper bag.

After putting my thumb on the card a dozen times a day for a week and seeing only black, I was sure of one thing. The card was broken. How could I—happy, bubbly, and sunny 99 percent of the time—be so stressed? And furthermore, how could I be so unaware?

To corroborate my *defective card theory*, I handed the card to my 11-year-old stepson, Crosby. He was wincing over math homework at the kitchen table, tapping his toe a mile a minute and scrunching his shoulders. Math was not his favorite subject.

"Put your thumb on this and count to ten," I quietly commanded. I was sure that I would see a big, fat, black square like mine.

"Here," he answered, handing the card back to me without looking up. The card had turned **blue**! *Yogi blue.*

"Are you kidding me?" I hollered to the sky. Apparently, Niravi was right. I was a basket case and didn't even know it.

Yet, my body did.

In my sessions with Niravi, I quickly discovered that beneath my authentic optimism steamed a simmering volcano of resentment, frustration, and anger. These reactions were the logical result of trying to please everyone all the time— everyone except myself. No wonder I felt selfish clinging to what seemed an impossible dream. Every doctor I ever met said that I was too sick to bear my own children.

How powerful are unconscious, negative beliefs?

They own us.

Though I had indeed come far, whenever we attempt to break through the glass ceiling of whatever we want most, we bump into old wounds again. At this moment, my glass ceiling was motherhood.

Niravi taught me 60-second meditations to relax my body and make the card turn blue. One might think that 37 years of stress—hospitalizations and physical and emotional trauma—would take eons to reverse. But in only one month, I began to reconnect my body to my brain. If I noticed myself sighing; if my neck was stiff; if Kenny and I were disagreeing; I would find a quiet space for meditation. And that card would turn blue. Sometimes, five minutes would pass instead of 60 seconds, but I began to trust the process. The human body and brain are miracles. That card wasn't broken after all— and neither was I.

I had ignited my inner healer, also known as the "Vital Force." Paul and Patricia Bragg wrote about Vital Force in the 1940s and 1950s, long before science validated the mind-body connection. They knew that stress was as toxic as pesticides in our food. Deep breathing to release stress and biofeedback have always been key components of the Bragg Healthy Lifestyle. No wonder Patricia Bragg radiates joy with fewer wrinkles than many 40-year-olds!

I began working with Niravi in April of 1992. At the end of August, I became pregnant. My acupuncturist sensed the pregnancy in my pulse a week before the home test read positive. I was elated and anxious. I felt pulled between the desire to join Kenny on the road and the physical challenges this presented—late nights, hotel food, and airport fumes. Keeping my promise to prioritize self-care, I canceled all travel. I had never done anything like that before. *Wasn't my role as Kenny's wife to be with him always? What will happen if I'm not there?* My fearful mind had a field day with that one. After all, I was married to a rock star!

"Not your problem—not your job," said a new voice inside.

Fighting demons and becoming aware of old patterns takes work. The battle was constant, scary, and uncomfortable. This new world looked and felt entirely unfamiliar. When the fear of another miscarriage or the repercussions of putting myself first would grip my chest, I would do my meditation. I was determined to liberate myself from a way of being that was no longer my own.

Daily I would say this mantra: "I am ready, willing, and able to release every limiting belief about myself and who I am in the world. I have no one to please except myself."

On May 22, 1993, Lukas Alushka Loggins came bravely into this world.

CHAPTER 2

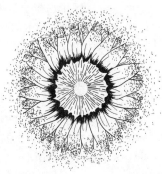

THE CARE PLAN

"Classic health is the true foundation on which every intelligent woman builds her vitality and beauty!"

—Patricia Bragg, Health Pioneer and Author

The goal of the Patricia Bragg and Julia Loggins CARE Plan:

Creating
Ageless
Renewable
Energy

"The CARE Plan" is written for you to experience self-care as joyful, easy, and fun. The plan works optimally by starting at the beginning and moving, step-by-step, through the program. However, you may dig into a module that attracts you and start there. You really cannot make a mistake. Each day is a new day.

"The CARE Plan" is a powerful process with the goal to renew whatever area calls your attention—energy, beauty, body, mind, and spirit. Start with what calls you. Birth is always accompanied by challenges. As you move through the modules, memories may appear, asking to be healed.

17

Be gentle with yourself. Ask for help. At this time in history, evolution has never been more conscious or supported. You are not alone. We rise together.

When you prioritize **you**—your health and happiness—you become instantly irresistible. As delicious as it feels to bathe in that attention, our hope is that you discover your life's purpose and revel in the rewards. Your limitless energy, crystal clear thinking, and newfound vitality multiply as you pour them into your passions. Revolutionary Beauties know that they are on this planet for a reason. Yet, we cannot maintain a high level of joy and focus without a Vital Nerve Force and a strong, healthy body free of pain, illness, and disease.

Thus, we start with the basics.

In this book, we will go through this journey together. We will heal the body, mind, and self-image with seven simple steps. We begin with the brain.

7 Steps to Create Ageless Renewable Energy (CARE)

1. Mindset: Healing the Brain and Tools to Release Unconscious Stress and Trauma

Releasing stress and trauma is the first step to regenerating the body and mind. As we liberate ourselves from negative, limiting beliefs, we discover how to embrace genuine self-acceptance. This allows us to practice "The CARE Plan" without force or self-sabotage. Stress is a part of life. Health issues, fatigue, and confusion are relieved by a Vital Nerve Force, the source of resilience and balance. We will help you fortify your nerve force with simple tools that grant you the ability to stand strong in a storm, stay present, and problem solve in a steady, relaxed manner. The tools we teach here build your Vital Nerve Force with simplicity and ease. This is the first secret of ageless beauty.

In this first module, we also address the limbic system, *the lookout tower* in the brain that alerts us when danger is present. When we've experienced trauma, stress, illness, or toxins, the limbic system is wounded, which results in overactive and hypervigilant reactions. This affects self-confidence, faith, and consistency with self-care. Through the steps outlined here, you will learn to identify the symptoms of a wounded limbic system. With the tools we offer, you may begin to heal. Now you are in the driver's seat, capable of carrying through on the practices you learn. You are no longer at the mercy of past situations.

As you begin, be as loving towards yourself as you would be with your child or a cherished friend. Every step is a step forward, even if you feel lost. Forgive yourself daily for what you did not know or could not do. Write the word "perfection" on a big poster board and use for dart practice! Scribble it on pieces of paper to throw in your fireplace and burn. Replace *perfect* with *I am enough*. There. Is. No. Going. Back. Every day is a new day. That's mother nature's law.

2. Purification: Detoxifying the Body

In 1970, Patricia authored *The Amazing New Hollywood Plan for Beautifying The Complexion and Body*, wherein she writes: "Classic health is the true foundation on which every intelligent woman builds her vitality and beauty! Vital cleanliness, through purification, is essential for a youthful face and body."

Detoxification is key to regeneration and energy. Contemporary research shows that today's humans connect with at least 2,500 chemicals daily. Yet, even before modern day toxins, the ancients understood the power of cleansing. You will learn uncomplicated, effective practices to cleanse your body. Transform your home into a spa, a sanctuary of renewal and calm as the foundation of your "CARE Plan." The simple tools taught here for colon cleansing, liver detoxification, lymphatic drainage, and breast health bring you renewable energy. With these basic practices to reboot renewal, you will find the optimism and happiness to enjoy life again. Your health and beauty are truly in your own hands.

Some of these cleansing practices may feel strange and unfamiliar. Yet, our great-great-grandmothers knew these secrets. Revolutionary Beauties remember who they are, and connect to the wisdom of their ancestors. If something feels uncomfortable, step back and circle around as you gain confidence. Just remember that the *norm* in society is a low bar of sickness, depression, and disease. When you stop buying that as your fate, you may indeed feel outside the norm. Don't let anyone tell you that *aging*, meaning *the end of youth* is inevitable.

If you're angry, that's okay. Anger is the gateway to action. In Tom Petty's words, "Everybody has to fight to be free." That's what Revolutionary Beauties do. They stand and fight, for the right to health and happiness, from which radical beauty flows. Welcome to the ring. Put on your golden gloves!

3. Liquid Nutrition and Intermittent Fasting

Fasting jump starts cell regeneration, stimulates metabolism, and rests digestion critical to creating renewable energy. "The CARE Plan" introduces three ways to fast. While you are on your healing journey, you will find a comfortable launching pad to integrate this amazing practice. One step leads to another. Each is a building block in creating ageless energy and beauty.

Organic vegetable juices, bone broths, and sugar-free protein shakes—what we call *liquid nutrition*—make fasting gentle and accessible. Liquid nutrition is key to eliminating cravings, reducing inflammation, balancing blood sugar, and elevating your mood.

The symptoms fasting may cause—headaches or fatigue—are due to the body's release of toxins into overwhelmed organs, the colon, and the liver. Picture pouring ten pounds of garbage into a garbage can already packed to the brim. Integrating the cleansing protocols from "Module 3" entirely reduces or eliminates these symptoms. Feel the lightness of your being and the mental clarity that comes with fasting. This blissful experience inspires the choice for clean and healthy food to synthesize this buoyant energy as your *new normal*.

4. The CARE Fueling Station and Food Combining:

Based on the Bragg Healthy Lifestyle, "The CARE Plan" is designed to make meals and snacks fast and easy to prepare—plus, delicious, nutritious, and fun!

"The CARE Fueling Plan" includes the basics of food combining, which is key to digestive health and to achieve and maintain a healthy weight, without deprivation. We teach you to monitor and create alkaline balance, heal candida or yeast overgrowth, tame your sweet tooth, and heal acid reflux—all keys to a happy gut.

Best-selling author and nutritionist Liana Werner-Gray shares 11 delicious, sugar, dairy, and gluten-free recipes in the Revolutionary Beauty Meal Plan. Her recipes were created for busy women with a full plate—notwithstanding what they are planning for dinner!

In this module, you will learn *crave control* through the use of digestive enzymes, improved absorption, and adequate protein consumption. Your cravings will no longer own you. You will gain control over hunger, moods, and blood sugar. This gives you freedom to make healthy choices, even during times of stress when you are prone to *emotional eating*.

5. Movement and Flexibility

Exercise and movement energize the body and calms the mind. Flexibility is key to longevity. Sensuality flows natural-ly from a body that moves fluidly and is pain-free. "The CARE Movement Guide" shares a variety of choices that bring a buoyant sense of being. We share the joys of dance and fit-ness, and we offer simple home routines. In the Resource Guide, you will find links to free classes and online resources.

"Module 5" describes the forms of yoga that include restor-ative yoga—a gentle practice perfect for those with limited physicality. We share the principles of Pilates, a detail orient-ed practice excellent and safe for anyone of any age. Our fit-ness experts share secrets for finding your personal fitness style, whether that is a brisk walk in the fresh air or shaking your booty in a Zumba dance class.

6. Hormones, Sensuality, and Pleasure

Confused about hormones, and their effect on your health and your mood? "The CARE Plan" explains the choices. Ver-ified by interviews with expert doctors, apply the informa-tion to make health decisions best for you.

In the second episode, we dive into the subject of sensuality and pleasure. Ageless beauties enjoy being in their bodies, no matter what size or age they are. Beauty and allure are determined by how we feel about ourselves. We offer sim-ple practices to help you explore your relationship with your body, to rediscover pleasure. Free yourself of the self-crit-icism of youth. Liberate yourself from comparisons to the retouched photos on social media. Enjoy sensual pleasure, with or without a partner, as simple self-delight.

Pleasure flows from the ability to receive. For many, that means to quiet the part of us that is focused on duty and doing for others. Many successful women—breadwinners, mothers, and partners—navigate the world through a high-ly developed masculine side. This compels them to perform no matter how they feel, or how heavy the load. This may render them unable to respond to their body's signals of ex-haustion and burnout—often because they don't feel them.

The beautiful feminine side is sadly neglected. Our inner Mother Nature—the source of life and *fountain of youth*—is capable of miracles. She is the womb of abundance, faith, renewal, love, and healing. Mother Nature holds dreams and attracts limitless opportunities. She opens doors, just through her magnetic energy. Her presence is enough, al-ways. She need not do a thing.

In this module, you will learn to tap into your inner *queen bee*. Queen bees know the survival of their tribe depends on their ability to receive—to allow the Universe to show up with exactly what they need.

If you're thinking, "If I don't do it, it won't get done," we hear you. However, we must challenge that belief system because the propensity for over-responsibility is killing us. We know that health and happiness, as well as desirability, depend on our dare. In this episode, we arm you with tools to trade sacrifice for self-worth, and to accomplish more than ever with half the effort. In one simple exercise, you will completely transform how you make decisions. Discover how and why you no longer must build the train, plus push that load up the mountain by yourself.

This module reconnects you to your discernment meter. Per-sonal boundaries make us feel safe to receive again. With what most women have experienced, the fact that they still stand is astonishing. But here you are. Your strength needs no proof. You have lived many lives in one. Time for joy. Time for faith. Time to look in the mirror and smile at yourself.

In this culture, that is revolutionary.

7. Skincare: Simplicity Redefined

"The CARE Skincare Plan" is based on five-minute per day rituals that stimulate collagen. This will improve skin texture, reduce lines, breakouts, and adult acne. We will teach you how to make your skin sparkle and glow. Turn the clock back twenty years or more! Yes, this is truly possible.

Our experts share the secrets of glowing skin and explain top-shelf protocols, methods, and practices—including lasers and peels. You will learn how to care for your skin. If confused about effectiveness and safety in the world of alternative and conventional skincare practices, this module offers the answers.

With "The CARE 5-Step Program," you will see the shine you thought disappeared through too little sleep and too much worry. You will learn strategies for peels you can do in your home to reduce fine lines, wrinkles, and puffy eyes. *Viva la Revolution, Beauty!*

After all your work to cleanse and heal your body, and recharge your energy, the reward is luminous, ageless skin. We will show you how!

In Patricia Bragg's words, "Woo-hoo! Here we go!"

MODULE 1

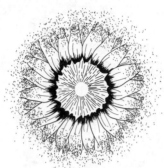

Episode 1
CREATIVITY & PURPOSE

"There are two great days in a person's life ...
The day we are born
And the day we discover why."

—William Barclay, Scottish Theologian and Author

Love in Action

At the core of Revolutionary Beauty is passion and purpose. Everyone asks, what is Patricia Bragg's beauty secret? This lifelong athlete played tennis and swam well into her seventies. At 92, her face looks decades younger. Her magic potion? She attributes her youthfulness solely to her lifestyle and work; plus a mission that launches her from bed at dawn like a rocket ship! Every morning she asks, "Who can I reach today? What needs to be done?"

You may think, "I have no idea what my purpose is. I'm too busy with life to even figure it out, much less make it happen." The good news is that your purpose will reveal itself as you become more in tune with your desires and creativity. It is that simple.

In their book, *Conscious Loving Ever After*, best-selling authors and ever-evolving creatives, Gay and Kathlyn Hendricks, PhD, write that the creative process starts with one statement: "I commit to enjoying my full capacity for love and creativity."

Say this out loud a few times. Gay and Kathlyn go on to say, "When you make a commitment to enjoying more love and creativity, you're saying to the world (and to yourself) that you intend to create joy, rather than suffering, in the two most important areas of your life."

When Gay and Kathlyn use the word "love," they do not refer to romantic love, but to the fertile imagination and energy that surges within us. Like a river, this love is infinite, wild, and untamed. Society does not dictate love's path. Pioneers and trailblazers are seldom embraced by the masses. Women, by nature, are trailblazers, eight-arm goddesses, spirits inhabiting flesh. Just as love is fierce, so are women.

The older we are, the more wisdom we acquire, and the more prepared we are to actively love, even if we take baby steps. To actively love ourselves is to treat the body like a temple. We honor ourselves with the bounty of the harvest, with silent meditation and the joy of song. We go to the temple to heal, to pray, to rest, and to dream of a brighter future.

That may feel odd at first. Only when we practice self-care are we replenished enough to take grand actions. Maybe we become activists. Maybe we turn the soil in our backyard into a garden. Maybe we share poetry with the community or write a book. Since statistics show most of us will be working well into our seventies, perhaps we start a business—one that leverages passions and skills we have learned along the way. Doesn't doing something we love make sense? One of the meaningful missions of self-care is to build the strength, stamina, and structure to transform dreams into reality. Needless ruminating and suffering over choices—or lack of them—is not Mother Nature's intent. This is the mandate and the manifesto of the Revolutionary Beauty. We were born for this moment.

The *Patricia Braggs* of the world shun retirement. More fascinating to them is to dive deeper into their message and hone it like a polished diamond. See the gleam in their eyes when they speak. Feel their playfulness and humility, as they do what they love most. When we hear role models like these tell their stories—their failures, their fumbles, and falls—we are encouraged to discover our own gifts. We each desire a life of meaning and fulfillment, beyond the worthy role of a loving partner, parent, daughter, or child. We deserve to take that first step toward making dreams a reality.

How can we not?

We may have survived turbulent childhoods, toxic environments, dangerous entanglements, divorce, illness, or bankruptcy. We may have lost everything only to come back stronger. We've raised kids, moved to a new life in a new city, and faced loss and heartbreak. We are still here. We have learned that we are well equipped to handle the unimaginable—good or bad. Discovering our strength, age leads us to learn why we are here, and let wisdom fuel, feed, and finally, fulfill us.

When we were young, people asked, "What do you want to be when you grow up?" We innocently answered from passion, no matter how impractical the dream. And we encouraged our children to reach for the sky, and let nothing hold them back. As the years rolled by, we may have stopped asking ourselves, "What do I want to be? What am I here for?" And yet, the question is as potent an inquiry at 40, 50, and 60 as it is at 18. We want to truly live, not just survive. And now, nontraditional ways to create income or to serve communities are at their greatest height.

"Where do we start?" we ask. We start with stories, day-dreams, and confessions to friends over hot cups of tea or glasses of wine. We scribble onto a napkin, or into a private journal. Use this module to tell your story. Discover your passion, and let these treasures lead you with conviction into the next chapter of your life.

At 4' 10", Patricia Bragg has never thought small or lived small. Let her be your guide as you birth your most exquisite self. Share exactly as you are called to do by your own inner compass.

Tell Your Story

Three years ago, I attended a stirring seminar on *the power of story*, given by former NFL star and Broadway playwright, Bo Eason. By asking each participant to share their three-minute story, we learned that nothing moves us more deeply than our own story. He stressed that vulnerability and transparency are keys telling to a riveting story. These autobiographical moments broke through stereotypes like a tornado blasting open hearts, and forever changed perceptions.

Bo says, "If you want to be successful at anything, you need to master the narrative of your life."

The story I shared was of a pivotal moment when a team of doctors informed me that I would not live beyond 17.

At 16—five months before my predicted death sentence—I nervously waited to see my 33rd doctor. Partially bald, with no eyebrows or eyelashes, weighing barely 100 pounds, I twitched nervously in my chair and prayed.

That fated day my new doctor—who would become my angel—initiated allergy testing as part of his solution. This involved injecting my arm with minuscule amounts of a food or pollen; then he monitored my body's vitals. Within minutes, my body reacted with anaphylactic shock, a life-threatening response to one of the allergens. I couldn't breathe and my throat swelled shut. This happened to me before, which necessitated many panic-stricken trips to the emergency room. This time was worse, and I passed out.

When I came back into my body, I felt a heavy painful thud. I looked into my doctor's eyes and saw his relief. He was crying. He said, "I'm right here. You're going to be OK."

My doctor had called 911. I know this because I was outside my body, watching him. As I peacefully floated above, for the first time I could recall, I felt no pain. I saw my doctor grab my hand; and he speak softly to me, "hold on." The paramedics arrived and applied electric shock pads to start my heart.

Just seconds prior, I had felt myself gliding through a tunnel. I saw light, and an unknown voice boomed: "It's not your time—you have work to do. Be assured this will never happen again, and you are not alone." In that tunnel, I knew from the core of my being that I would survive. And although years of healing were ahead, the 911 emergencies stopped. As I returned to consciousness, with the doctor holding my hand, I felt I could trust him. Together we would cheat the prognosis of my death before I reached 17. And we did.

With Bo's support, each member of the audience jumped on stage to tell their story. One of the country's most successful investors shared a childhood memory of dashing expectantly into the living room on Christmas morning, only find no presents under the tree. Her single mother barely had enough money with which to pay the light bill, let alone buy gifts. I felt the intensity of her promise to make something of her life and instantly knew why so many trusted her with their money. She understood the reality of having none. I learned more about her in those three minutes than I might have learned in an entire financial presentation.

Gifts are often hidden in stories, in the fabric of days we think we will not survive. Unexpectedly, we are called to make decisions or take actions that are fundamental to who we become. With backs against the wall, we may not feel the least bit heroic at the time. The choice is to either quit, give up, or dig in. How did we find that last shred of courage? Sharing your story creates instant credibility and true connection.

Your story may be one you have not yet discerned which makes you uniquely valuable. You may say, "I just did what had to be done—what anyone would do." Nevertheless, when you tell your story, look straight into the eyes of the listener. Witness your strength reflected in their awe.

The other day a young client I'll call Leila asked me for advice in creating a flyer for her new career as a private chef. The fee Leila was about to charge was way below the going rate. I asked her why.

"Oh, I'd do this for free," she exclaimed, barely containing her excitement. "I adore helping people eat a cleaner diet, organize their pantry, and even plant a garden. So many people freeze when they get into their kitchen. I love teaching them that cooking is easy and fun. The best feeling in the world is when clients tell me I've changed their life."

She told me this as if cooking was the simplest thing in the world, something anyone can do. I asked her to share what originally inspired her career. Leila answered, "When I was ten, I was playing at my best friend's house. Her mom asked if we wanted to help make a salad. She had all kinds of fresh vegetables on the counter, food I had never seen. She let me taste every single one. I'll never forget that first bite of cucumber! We rarely ate salad at my house. My mom worked two jobs and served us TV dinners or boxed mac and cheese. That afternoon was amazing! My friend's mom was so warm and friendly. I thought, 'I want to go to people's houses and make yummy food for them! How fun would that be?'"

"I didn't think I could afford culinary school. Thanks to my local college who offered the course for free, here I am!"

Leila's story brought me to tears. I could see the passion in her eyes and feel the satisfaction her work brings. No wonder she's changing people's lives.

What is your life changing moment? Trust whatever comes to mind. That experience may not have been immediately transformative. Your fork in the road might have been inspired by your most embarrassing incident. Perhaps you have a handful of instances that qualify. We often do. We are given glimpses of our purpose throughout life. Sometimes we notice, and sometimes we do not. The story you write may not instantly reveal your sacred skill, but can potentially galvanize an inquiry you had not considered.

Take an hour—not more—to write a three-minute story describing your life changing moment. Be sure to describe the thoughts, feelings, and conclusions this experience inspired. Do this exercise a dozen times, and you will learn something new every time.

Read your story aloud to yourself a few times, over the course of a week. Listen for subtle meanings and metaphors. Detect shifts in your body or messages from your dreams.

Patricia Bragg adores telling personal stories to bring to life the principles for which she stands, making them accessible. When someone is transparent, dismissing them is nearly impossible. And, by the way, stumbling is inevitable. Most of us are so focused on perfection we forget that our clumsiest moments are the most endearing. If you ask your best friend or partner what they love about you, they will probably tell a funny story about the quirky side of you that only they have seen.

Be prepared to be completely astonished by the story you have chosen. Don't censor or second-guess your imagination.

Discover Your Passion

In their New York Times Best Seller, *The Passion Test*, Janet Attwood, and Chris Attwood offer thought-provoking tools to discover your passions and build a life around them.

One of their first suggestions in boosting creativity is to "Resign as the *General Manager of the Universe*." For those of us who were burdened with unreliable support systems, this is not easy and can feel terrifying. However, letting go of the need to control the environment—and everyone around us—opens up an entire world of time and energy. The mantra "I no longer need to control my environment to feel safe" is a wonderful way to begin the process.

Their next suggestion is to list the pursuits that interest you. Then, shrink that list to your top five. This intriguing exercise allows your inner wisdom to reimagine your future. Take an hour to write your first list. Take as much time as you need to select top five that give you chills and goosebumps.

Warning: Expect immediate resistance. Your mind will shout the fifty ways you'll never make a living doing what you love—or find your purpose or soul mate. Remember, the mind is simply a storehouse of experiences—not the birthplace of imagination. Now, we must take control and reorganize that warehouse. Without denying or negating trials and tribulations, this next part of life will be lived heart first. Lean into new ideas and experiences that bring joy.

Living in the Zone

Do you recall a time when you felt you were *in the zone?* A client, Roxanne, recently did this exercise. To her surprise, "being with kids," surfaced as her number one passion. At 64, her own children were grown and lived far away. Furloughed from her job, and trepidatious as to what her future might hold, this revelation gave her an idea for a new career.

Roxanne took a CPR class. She registered with a local child-care agency and is now a nanny to two little girls.

Roxanne sent me this note: "I am so happy! The girls squeal when I walk in the door. Their giggles make me smile non-stop. We play. We do silly things. We dig in the garden and read. I cook with them, and now they love salads. Their dad tells me that is a first. I've been helping their mom with book-keeping. Every mother needs a village! This lovely job fills my heart and pays my rent. I'm so grateful. I wish I'd started this career years ago."

Another client, Elaine, was surprised that her number one choice was painting—a passion she had walked away from twenty years ago because her parents admonished that her art would never pay the bills. This is her story.

"So, I did that list that you suggested. After that, could I re-sist picking up a brush again? No. I invested $75 in paint. I cre-ated an ocean mural with dolphins and colorful tropical fish on the inside of my garage, just for fun. I loved the activity so much that I had to remind myself to stop and eat. When my husband's boss and wife arrived for dinner, they spotted my mural and couldn't stop complimenting my art. As a result, they hired me to create a mural for their son's room. This assignment led to another commission, and then another. I just quit my job at the bank and I'm now painting full-time. Who would have thought?"

Sacred Selfishness

The number one goal of creativity is happiness. The exhilara-tion of fulfilling our destiny soothes and satisfies the soul in a way nothing else can. Though purpose may compel you to *work* twenty hours a day, you will feel energized. Trust that your mind and body are ready, willing, and able to support this journey.

When we have experienced betrayal, rebuilding self-trust can take years. I've known women who have forgiven each hurtful person in their lives but have not forgiven themselves for the choices they have made. If you are blaming yourself for past lifestyle choices, take a big breath of forgiveness and compassion. You deserve peace, harmony, and happiness. You have the right to discover your purpose and feel the joy and satisfaction of a life truly lived.

Purpose minimizes the pain of just about everything. Shifts in personal lives and uncontrollable world events are neutralized by grounded creativity. In the most gratifying way, we become deeply focused. When we're *in the zone*, completely engrossed, mundane troubles melt into the background. We return to daily life, filled with a sense of presence and mastery.

Each word of this book was written so that you could experience this coveted place, pain-free, and full of energy. Spending my childhood in the hospital taught me that joy can be unfamiliar territory when crisis is the norm. I learned to savor each day. If we are sick or hurt, or someone close to us is suffering, then, we circle the wagons. We take whatever measures are necessary to ensure the path to wellness. Without hesitation, we take action and ask for help. When all is well, we reenter life in celebration and gratitude.

When I was at Hippocrates, where many people came to heal life-threatening disease, I observed patients who left with a clean bill of health. Yet, they spent the rest of their lives living in fear that their cancer would return or their partner would relapse.

If you are burned-out from going nonstop since you learned to walk, consider that your first act of sacred selfishness may be to stop and rest. Most people don't have the ability to leave jobs and families and check into a health spa for a month. *Rest* means assessing your level of exhaustion—

possibly with the support of a skilled health practitioner—and following orders, plus hearing your inner wisdom. Asking for help is a challenge for women. Do you ever say, "I'm done. I need a break?" But, when we don't take that break, we break. And, when we hit *the wall*, renewing ourselves takes precious time and energy.

Creating Dreamtime

The next step in "sacred selfishness" is to create weekly dreamtime. That is a period of at least twenty minutes when you gaze at the clouds or sit quietly in a park and dream. Conscious dreamtime is an undervalued and neglected luxury from which groundbreaking ideas and inventions spring. "The Nap Ministry" is a new movement that promotes *rest as resistance*. Dreamtime is a rebellion against the *grind culture*, a society that glorifies constant striving, regardless of the physical and mental cost. *Walden; Or, Life in the Woods* author Henry David Thoreau would be proud.

Mary Oliver gives us this quote from her poem, "The Summer Day,"

> I don't know exactly what a prayer is
> I do know how to pay attention, how to fall down into
>   the grass, how to kneel in the grass.
> How to be idle and blessed, how to stroll through the
>   fields,
> Which is what I have been doing all day.
> Tell me, what else should I have done?
> Doesn't everything die at last, and too soon?
> Tell me, what is it you plan to do
> With your one wild and precious life?

Dreamtime sits patiently waiting until the mind is finally quiet and the spirit surveys the horizon. Solo time is as vital as clean food, exercise, and deep breathing.

When you are alone, be conscious of your self-talk. Speak to yourself the way you would a beloved child. With no clock ticking on personal evolution, take time to discover your passions. No one is measuring your progress.

Manifest Your Dream

Before spending time and money on a new project, run your idea by one or two trustworthy confidantes. Choose people invested in your success, but also willing to tell the truth. I discovered late in life that I rarely confided in those close to me, for fear they would squash my dreams. I can see now that blundering ahead—while I felt good at the time—sometimes squandered precious time and resources.

This is a pattern many women share. We are accustomed to being unsupported. We guard our dreams like mother bears. My fountain of ideas is inspiring, yet not all of them deserve to see the light of day. I'm grateful to my husband for his clear-eyed, openhearted opinions. His only agenda for me is to be happy and successful. In addition, he is willing to share me with my purpose.

When we first met, his mature self-sufficiency was unfamiliar. He did not need me to cook his dinner or worry about his workload—and found my desire to do so unattractive! As a former all-star codependent, I questioned how to use the extra time away from work and children, if not to take care of him. When I explained my quandary he said, "Well, you've always wanted to write a book. Do it!"

So, with his encouragement, I wrote one, and then another. He and my children shared me with my computer for hundreds of hours while I worked around the clock at the kitchen table. They never complained. They didn't create emotional dramas. I learned that by watching me do what I love, my family began to do the same. We cheered for each other. My daughter wrote a novel. My son became an incredible chef and finished a degree in sustainable agriculture. My husband retired from a company he built and is constructing the next chapter of his life. That's what we want for our beloveds— their genuine happiness and fulfillment.

Renew, Regenerate, Rest, Risk, Repeat

This is only the beginning. As you know, healing, growing, and reinventing life does not happen linearly. The dance of *renew, regenerate, rest, risk, repeat* heals bodies, minds, and spirits. As we heal, we're able to fully embrace joy and creativity. When we do, we glow from the inside with a light that will not be dimmed. This is the recipe for ageless beauty.

Revolutionary Beauty celebrates radical change and a paradigm shift from "disposable to renewable." Patricia Bragg has fought for this mindset all her life. Yet, she does not consider her beliefs radical, just practical. The idea that poison doesn't belong in our bodies—or in the soil, water, or air— and that we deserve to be happy and healthy, is a simple, straightforward concept. At this moment in time, however, it is revolutionary.

At times, rest is more valuable than taking action. Fasting can be more healing than eating. These are principles as ancient as the *Dead Sea Scrolls*. In fact, these understandings of how to regenerate body and spirit are found painted on cave walls, pottery, and in temples and churches worldwide. Indeed, the quote, "What has been done will be done again; there is nothing new under the sun," applies to cleansing practices. So, let's remember and value the origins of the ancient purification rituals.

Healing and reclaiming joy and power is our birthright. No one can take that journey for us. However, we each follow an inner road map—our North Star. If you are reading this book, you have never been more ready. As Patricia Bragg says, "You are the captain of your own ship!"

Patricia always knew her worth. She knew the value of her mission. Though financial abundance was never her focus, *The Queen of Natural Living* understood that what came naturally to her was a gift. The world rewarded her. When she speaks, she emphasizes the importance of individual contributions, and the impact they have.

Patricia is the ultimate champion—a premier motivational speaker long before the term was coined. The first question she asked when we met was, were my books as successful as they could be? (*Patricia Bragg is not shy.*) She wasn't talking about money. She was talking about value. What she really meant was, *did I grasp the urgency and importance of my message?* She did. She knew that was the foundation of success.

Don't wait for *the perfect day* to begin. As Patricia would say, "if you're lucky enough to be alive, today is perfect." You are the seeds, the soil, and the sun.

May you bloom with all the colors of the rainbow!

Revolutionary Beauty Lisa Proctor-Hawkins

Meet Lisa Proctor-Hawkins, brand strategist for brands that spark change and founder of Firefly180 Marketing.

Lisa: *For me, revolution evokes the word "revelatory," the willingness to reveal who you truly are. This lifelong process of peeling back our layers is our greatest challenge and like an unfolding rose, our most beautiful offering.*

Revolutionary Beauty is about understanding what are you here on this planet to do. A big part of that for me professionally has been to align mission with message—and as a former journalist and current brand and marketing strategist, I've been passionate about educating, activating, and empowering consumers to create positive change for more than 30 years.

In my personal life, there was a time when I believed love meant suffering for someone else. And in my younger years, I got a PhD in Martyrdom. It took me decades to realize that this did not serve me and it held others back.

My older, wiser, most beautiful self has no fear of death, but an absolute terror of not living. And I am more fully alive (physically, emotionally, and sexually) in my sixties than I have ever been. The key that has unlocked it all has been self-love. I had no idea how much I could love all the light and shadowy parts of me; but as I do, my heart continues to expand to love more and be loved even more. Nothing could be more beautiful!

MODULE 1

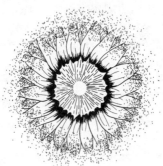

Episode 2
MIND OVER MATTER

*"The feminine essence waltzes with time.
Agelessness is power."*

—Julia Loggins, Digestive Health Expert and Author

When we refuse to buy society's definition of our self-worth, we reclaim power. Who, then, defines beauty? We do. First, we must face the demons that influence us to deny our self-worth and sparkle. Feeing beautiful is nearly impossible when wrestling with the demons of chronic pain, depression, and disease.

As Patricia would say, "Your health is your wealth," and must be your focus. The rewards are a strong body, an undeniable sensuality, and a road map to your destiny. Nothing makes us more beautiful than manifesting our best life.

Embarking on this plan, this *heroine's journey*, allows us to reclaim trust in ourselves. We build a bridge to connect head and heart and embody everlasting charisma. Challenging circumstances no longer derail us; they are opportunities to hone what we have learned. We become stronger, softer, and more vulnerable, and connect more deeply with each other. This is how we voice our separate identities. To heal a fragile planet that is desperate for us to awaken, we must love with ferocity and vision.

If reading this book, you are ready to become the most beautiful version of yourself.

Does this level of higher confidence seem unimaginable? True enough, some days we sparkle more than other days. If you could awaken pain-free, and filled with assurance that whatever comes your way, you will survive and thrive, imagine how different life would feel!

We are born to feel more attractive as we age. Designed to experience the last third of life as the icing on the (sugar-free) cake, this is when we create a legacy and revel in an unconditionally loving community. We find that community, our tribe, by first finding ourselves.

Revolutionary Beauties are not perfect or bulletproof, but have dropped defenses in exchange for exquisite discernment—the choice to construct boundaries rather than walls. If the question before you is complex, the right answer may not reveal itself for a week or a month. There's no rush. The feminine essence waltzes with time. Agelessness is power. What gives us patience and resilience is the creation of what Patricia Bragg calls a powerful "Vital Force," a strong nervous system that withstands the storms of our lives while supporting the re-creation of a new way of being. Slowing down is one of the Revolutionary Beauty's secrets to life.

We are moving at rocket speed and doing the impossible. Women are eight-arm goddesses—balancing career with family life, community responsibilities, and often, caring for parents, children, or grandchildren. With an evergrowing to-do list, slowing down seems counterintuitive. But, this is the best place to start, and it may be a preeminent gift that you ever give yourself. When we resist slowing down, we lose our ability to discern and we weaken our boundaries. Not only do we lose our sense of beauty, but our insecurities also take over. And nothing else ages us faster.

Beauty invites us to embrace the sensuality of each moment. Imagine dining at the finest restaurant in Paris for a five course feast, and feeling pressure to consume the cuisine in an hour. Rather than relishing each bite, basking in the elegant decor, swooning over the dessert tray, we shove food in our mouths without savoring. That is how many of us life live. To move this quickly taxes our nervous system, twists the gut, and ages skin. Generally, this happens without awareness on our part. We've been operating full tilt for so long, we cannot imagine another way to be.

For Revolutionary Beauties, self-care takes precedence. This is not a self-serving choice, but rather a practical way to preserve the tribe's most precious asset: us. Without prioritizing ourselves, we draw on reserves soon depleted, which leaves us empty and frustrated. This stirs drama and destroys our self-worth.

Do you remember the movie, *The Princess Diaries*? In the film, Mia, a shy, awkward California teenager (played by Anne Hathaway) learns that she is heir to the throne of a European kingdom. Under the tutelage of the reigning queen, her grandmother (played by Julie Andrews), Mia sheds insecurity and steps and into womanhood. By the end of the movie, Mia fully embodies her new role as the elegant—and lighthearted—ruler of the fictional country of Genovia. Retold by Hollywood, it is a timeless fairy tale. In patriarchal mythology, birth order decides who will be queen. In today's new feminine mythology, we make that decision.

Today, you inherit a kingdom. Your mind and body are the crown jewels. This is the moment to commit to your health and happiness.

Care for your castle with tenacity, commitment, compassion, and humor. Loving our bodies and reclaiming beauty and power is a lifelong journey. Through Mother Nature's wisdom, you will liberate yourself from toxins that bind, and reclaim your birthright of unchained happiness.

That's Patricia Bragg's power style. Her *Declaration of Independence* springs from living the truth she knows. This book will help you write your own unique *Declaration of Independence*. Before you know it, this manifesto will have changed you. With this vision, you can change the world.

You will step into Patricia's universe, and you will never be the same.

Action Steps

1. Remember a time you felt truly beautiful. Whether you were a child, playing dress-up in your mother's clothes and posing gleefully in front of the mirror, or as a teen, draped in a prom gown, or even in your dreams. Take a moment and, engaging all of your senses, soak in this scene. Bask in the liberation and exhilaration. Now write in these next pages some of the descriptive words about what you're feeling. Peaceful? Powerful? Thankful? Whole? Allow yourself to come back here at any time.
2. Dig knee-deep into the rich soil of your inner garden. Imagine how you would feel doing exactly what you love to do. Is that being free to play outside all day with your children, writing alone, or perhaps even baking? Write in your journal what you would love to do if you could allow yourself to find a way. Now, you have a reminder of how to recharge your batteries.
3. When we are with our partners, family, or friends, do we give them our full attention? Do we truly listen? Most importantly, do we give ourselves time to daydream, journal, or sit in a park and just look at the sky?

When I do, I am so replenished! This costs nothing, and yet, yields a treasure. Today, as you take your first step onto the path to attaining Revolutionary Beauty, slow down. Take a breath. Review your to-do list. What can you delegate? What and who really needs your attention? Can you cross off anything from the list?

Once, when I had moved, somehow, the post office confused my forwarding address and my mail did not reach me for three months. By the time I opened my mail, I calculated that 75 percent had become irrelevant and the other 25 percent was handled in less than an hour. What a lesson!

Revolutionary Beauty Tracey Magill

Meet Revolutionary Beauty, Tracey Magill, former model, and CEO of Mindscape Industries, who reinvented her life at 56. Yet, if you laid eyes on Tracey, you would swear she is not a day over 35. As she says, "My script is being rewritten."

Tracey: *Marrying my first boyfriend from high school, a five-year engagement was a recipe for disaster. It was a tumultuous marriage; my husband had a strong, willful personality just as the men from my childhood. I filed for divorce, lost my home through his embezzlement of my savings, entered a homeless shelter with my child. I survived, fought my way out. I was 27.*

A second marriage lasting twenty-two years followed, and a second son was born. During this cycle, I electively blew my life up, leaving behind money, power, and everything else in order to save my soul. My first therapy session began. I also sought spiritual healing on a deeper level. I had come to believe in a higher force or creator in a different manner. A force that does not judge or demand. That does not give us too much to handle, just enough in order to learn.

Therapy took me to the core of comprehending the choices I had made and why. There were days I would leave the therapist's office drained, numb, and exhausted. I was an onion peeling back layers, week after week to reach the center. Upon doing so, another cycle began. This cycle equipped me with a tool belt attached at the hip. It is natural and organic for me to nurture the well-being of others. However, with my newfound tool belt, I have the capability to remain detached while extending kindness, compassion, and guidance to all; allowing my sons to fall while observing from the wings, as opposed to enabling and saving, refraining from creating one better situation than the last for them. This planet is a classroom to learn and grow, I would not be much help as a mother to their growth if I enabled it. The old script would have permitted the opposite, but not today.

Through past circumstances, reaching 50 is truly when my life's journey began. With a staff force of 250, and as CEO and founder I stood in my power feeling free.

Fifty-five brought a new tool to my belt, Julia Loggins. Life had taken its toll on my health, I was dying on the inside, the factory was tired. Julia saved my life. It is my body, the façade that houses my soul, therefore the responsibility falls upon me to nurture it. With Julia's guidance, I am able to maintain a healthy gut, resulting in the obliteration of a protruding tummy, continuous constipation, inflammation, etc. Through dedication, my body has morphed strong and lean while my skin radiates health and an inner glow. My body is happy. Julia completed my tool belt.

I am alive, vibrant, empowered, blooming, clear, and stronger than ever before at 56. Viewing life in the present, eager to move along, excited to embrace the next cycle and where it may take me. Peace, joy, and harmony are top of my list. I can navigate with ease to the delete button, iron out any creases that may rumple the page. I am not a victim, I am a survivor, I remain in my truth. My script has been rewritten allowing life's lessons to unleash a Revolutionary Beauty that has a wingspan so vibrant it is infectious.

MODULE 1

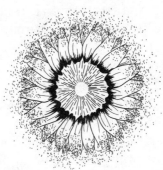

Episode 3
STRESS, TRAUMA
& THE LIMBIC SYSTEM

"A highly influential, walnut-sized area—deep in the center of your brain—is live wired with functions critical to survival. The limbic system in your brain, in fact, influences problem solving, organization, and rational thought, among other things."

—Dr. Daniel Amen, Psychiatrist and Founder of Amen Clinics

As an environmentally sensitive, wheezy, inhaler carrying kid, more than one doctor said to me, "Julia, it's all in your head." At the time, I speculated, *are they right?* I felt humiliated, ashamed, and helpless. I would have done anything to change my condition. And, for the last four decades, I've witnessed the anguish of clients struggling with the same question. In the words of Anaïs Nin, "We don't see things as they are. We see things as *we* are."

My clients did not create their illness, nor did I. And, you did not create yours. No one wants to be sick or in pain. Physical conditions are real. Childhood patterns and belief systems contribute to the manifestation of physical conditions—as do genetics, toxins, stress, and brain injuries.

My limbic system injury not only perpetuated health issues, but it also triggered my beauty-wound—in fact, it was a foundational aspect of its creation. Until I identified and healed this part of my brain, I rarely felt *good enough*. I struggled to determine the difference between real danger and imagined threats in every part of my life—a setup for frequent misinterpretations and inner turmoil.

A poem I wrote for *Unimaginable Life*, called "Your Spirit and My Spirit," describes this slippery slope. Here is a piece of it:

> So what if I make you
> Mashed potatoes and real gravy
> Because you love it
> Pick up my bathroom towels
> So what if I wear a dress and curl my hair
> And you say I'm pretty, and I wonder,
> Is this me, is this real
> Is this honest, is this safe
> Holding tightly onto my sound bites of self-respect
> To use on you like an Uzi.

Chronic Pain Loops

Forty years ago, a groundbreaking discovery determined that all trauma—physical, emotional, and mental—changes the way the neural pathways work in the brain. These injuries can lead to the creation of chronic pain loops, such as fibromyalgia, and environmental sensitivities. Symptoms include a host of mental and emotional disorders that ravage the immune system and shred nerves: post-traumatic stress disorder (PTSD), anxiety, and depression. In other words, high stress is brain poison. So, in a way, doctors were right. *Something was wrong in my head.* However, limbic system injuries were unknown as I fought for my life as a kid in ICU.

The understanding of *neuroplasticity*—the fact that the brain *can* heal—is the biggest news in science since Galileo discovered that the world was round. Dr. Michael Merzenich, in his book, *Soft-Wired*, calls the application of neuroplasticity "a revolution in the understanding of our humanity." Dr. Merzenich was one of the first scientists who introduced the concept that something beyond physical contact—like getting hit in the head—could cause a brain injury.

The limbic system is the *first responder* of the brain. Acting as the *lookout tower*, a healthy limbic system reads sensory input and interprets the difference between real and perceived threats. This part of the brain regulates the function of the parasympathetic and sympathetic nervous systems, which includes breathing, blood pressure, and response to emotional situations. Trauma can distort the limbic system's ability to correctly translate what is seen and experienced. These reactions are triggered by toxic exposure, accidents, sexual abuse, or any violent episode. Sustained periods of stress, a traumatic event, and long-term or acute illness can also trigger a false limbic system response. A perfect storm gathers when traumas occur at the same time, and the limbic system is pushed beyond its breaking point.

Two truths coexist. One is the well-known fact that the environmental chemicals used in farming and the foods they produce are a real threat to health. The other truth is less known. Since the limbic system responds to chemical sensitivities, people with a history of life-threatening symptoms react when they believe they have contacted a toxic substance. This is similar to a veteran with PTSD going into shock when they hear a loud sound on a video game. To them, the shock is real because the original trauma was real. When we're discussing PTSD, no one would say that feeling terror and shaking is an aberrant reaction to being in a war zone. The fight or flight message of "911! Your life is at risk," is the limbic system performing correctly. An injured limbic system sounds the alarm whether or not the danger is real.

Human DNA was designed to record danger and protect us from life-threatening situations. A wounded limbic system, however, keeps us from living in the present. Anything that remotely resembles a painful past experience is seen as a hazardous situation. The wound triggers the nervous system to respond as if the peril is present and real. As time passes, less stimulation is required to cause symptoms that feel or may be life-threatening.

This reaction is so unconscious and involuntary that we are left unaware. Thus, talk therapy doesn't always heal limbic system injuries. Those of us with wounded limbic systems are stuck in a repeating loop of constant stress. Some of us have extreme sensitivity to light or electromagnetic fields. Others are triggered by sound, smell, taste, touch—anything that replays the original trauma.

If this sounds familiar to you, you are not crazy! The good news is that brain injuries can heal. Most of the clients I have seen over the last 40 years who have dealt with chronic pain, addiction, eating disorders, or autoimmune disease experienced limbic system injuries. By the way, limbic system injuries are connected to digestive issues. We can learn how to retrain the brain so that symptoms no longer rule our lives. The power is in your hands. We're going to use that power to manifest health and happiness, starting right now.

How to Identify a Limbic System Injury

The following list of symptoms indicate that you may be experiencing a limbic system injury:

- Sexual abuse
- Chronic stress
- Chronic fatigue
- Disordered eating
- Survivor of violence

- Post-accident trauma
- Chronic pain, including fibromyalgia
- Food or substance addiction or abusive relationships
- Illness or injury—physical or psychological—not fully responding to traditional therapies and treatments
- Chemical sensitivities, such as reactions to perfumes, cosmetics, household cleaners, and preservatives

Chronic stress can damage the limbic system as intensely as any other trauma. Research has shown that chronic stress diminishes memory and the ability to release fearful experiences and *move on*. We begin to live in survival mode. More and more stress hormones flood the nervous system, which in turn validates hypervigilent behavior. The brain tells us that this type of behavior is a logical reaction to the environment. However, the limbic system wound is interpreting what is seen through fear.

Who does their best problem solving when panic-stricken, hyperventilating, and shaking? No one! We best problem solve when calm, breathing slowly, and in touch with innate intelligence, which equals gut instincts. The best medic in a situation is always the calmest. For a hypervigilant person who regularly scouts for a crisis, health and happiness must take a back seat. This way of being twists the gut into a knot, hijacks hormones, and cripples creativity.

The tricky thing about limbic system injuries is that the injury itself keeps us from identifying the injury. If you're in a car accident, you know when your neck hurts that you might have whiplash, and don't hesitate to avail yourself of treatment. But, limbic system injuries easily go unnoticed.

If you see your dilemmas in the following list, consider the possibility that you have a limbic system injury. Seek assistance to help you heal, as though you had a physical injury, such as whiplash.

- Resistance to getting help
- Inability to access joy and happiness
- Surviving childhood trauma of any kind
- Self-sabotage in relationships or at work
- Inability to complete proactive, self-help programs
- Difficulty manifesting or even identifying your goals
- Difficulty during transitions: hormonal changes, loss, or uncertainty

Happiness Matters

For those of us who have experienced trauma, especially in childhood, feelings such as joy, stability, acceptance, and enthusiasm can prompt uncomfortable physical and emotional sensations. We may find ourselves panting, squirming, or going numb when receiving a compliment. How do you feel when someone says, "You look beautiful today?" Do you recoil and say, "Oh, my god, my hair is a mess!" Or, "Thank you," and allow yourself to accept the compliment. The goal is to retrain the brain to value positive and happy thoughts.

Positive feelings are foreign to the part of us that was conditioned to stay small, not take up space, or make a mistake. We may feel if we spread our wings, we will get sent to our room at any moment—even if we're 35 or 55! A negative response can initiate from painful sensory memories all too familiar and now at play. A loving relationship or a well paying job with coworkers who think the world of us feels strange and untrustworthy.

"When will they see the real me?" we ask ourselves, waiting for the axe to fall.

A rewired brain is able to accept pleasure, treasure happiness, and value the feeling of steady ground. Only then can we build a solid foundation where self-acceptance thrives.

When I was introduced to the Hoffman Process, a step-by-step protocol for releasing emotional pain, I came face-to-face with an overwhelming amount of grief, sadness, and anger held in my body. These were feelings of which I was unaware—the result of unspoken traumas. Traumas, by the way, are not defined by their gravity. For example, not being validated as a person can be as devastating as a terrible car accident. The repeating loop of negative, painful, or fearful responses is the same for either trauma.

The tools I used to release the unconscious emotional pain that my body held allowed me to wrap my arms and heart around the hurt inner child. I wasn't going to let anyone hurt her again. I realized that although I wasn't perfect, I was a good person who deserved a life of joy. That awareness lit an inexhaustible fire that fueled my healing journey. Otherwise, I could not have chugged green juice three times a day for a year without regular donut binges—even if my life depended on this level of discipline—which it did. That commitment to my inner child shifted my attitude from silent victim to fierce protector.

At the time, I did not grasp the potency of that recognition. Why can some people stick to a healing program, while others struggle—and brutally punish themselves for what they perceive is a lack of willpower? The truth is that consistent self-care has little to do with willpower, and everything to do with self-love. Healing the mind and learning to release stress is the first step of any wellness and beauty program. Nothing is more toxic than stress. Stress toxins ruins the skin and steals our joy, whether internal or external. Trade those expensive face creams for time and space to meditate, purify your body, and eat natural food. The only thing Patricia Bragg uses on her face is olive oil!

The incredible truth is that no matter how old or young we are, our brains heal from within. The brain activity transforms from cinemas playing our worst moments to brilliant, problem-solving command centers, capable of anything.

In the movie, *Legally Blonde*, Reese Witherspoon plays a woman who discovers her power while pursuing a law degree from Harvard. In the last scene, she takes over the defense in a murder trial after her lascivious boss is fired. She wins the case by deducing a prosecutor's *shower alibi* was false—because everyone knows *women do not shower after getting a perm*. Meeting the press, she slyly delivers the line, "The rules of hair care are simple and finite. Any Cosmo Girl would have known."

That line always stuck with me. Number one, I always wanted to be a Cosmo Girl. (*Talk about compete and compare!*) The second is because the theme—what is real is obvious and simple—resonated deeply. The practices to heal our brain and body are astonishingly simple, as is everything authentic. As we heal the brain and release stress, the Vital Force ignites, which rejuvenates bodies, revitalizes dreams, and recaptures youthful optimism. As Patricia Bragg says, "This allows us to become the captains of our own ship."

If I can heal, so can you. You can heal even if—at this moment—you cannot get through the day without coffee and a donut. When you learn how to release the stress and trauma that is the source of cravings, the desire is dramatically reduced. One day, cravings disappear. We rebuild identity and sense of self from the inside out. We detoxify, from head to toe, which eliminates the hungry ghosts that therapy cannot liberate. As a result, we self-create irrefutable, ageless, and irresistible beauty. We own and deserve that transformation. Mother Nature has renewed even the most devastating forests after a fire, and the barest plains after a flood. The body, mind, and spirit are no different.

Patricia has been asked a thousand times how she eschewed meat, coffee, and even aspirin all these years. With a huge grin, she responds, "Because I know those things are bad for me, my dear! And, I have work to do. I love to awaken feeling good. My body deserves healthy food. Why would I do anything else?"

To be honest, I've known famous health advocates who secretly binged on Oreos and found solace at McDonald's in the middle of the night. But not Patricia. Her company was successful because every cell of her body lives and breathes her message—that everyone deserves to radiate health, happiness, joy, and beauty. She *worked her tush off* to build Bragg Live Food, which was effortless for her. The reason for her success is that her goal was never solely to make money. Her mission was to deliver healthy living to the world. There were no inconsistencies between thought and action to cause her to sabotage her success.

She never went to war with negative limiting belief systems. The definition of willpower is forcing ourselves to do what we know is right when our minds are telling us we cannot. The ensuing conflict spurs the flight or fight sensation which removes us from the present and invites fear, anger, frustration, and self-loathing. Biofeedback, meditation, journaling, and other brain training techniques release stress and elevate mood. These also regenerate our organs, skin (the largest organ in our body), hormones, and energy.

Paul Bragg and Patricia Bragg embraced a similar theme over 50 years ago in their book, *Nerve Force!* They taught that indifference, indecision, doubt, worry, and ill health were due to low energy, or low "Nerve Force." They write, "These two states—the physical and the mental—are so closely interrelated that it is impossible to separate them."

"Nerve Force," they continue, "is the most precious gift of Mother Nature. It is the Vital Force of life, a mysterious energy that flows from the nervous system to give life and energy to each vital organ.

It is responsible for everything: your happiness, your health, and your success in life. You must learn all there is to know about your nerves: how to protect, relax, calm, and soothe your nerves. Nerve Force is the dominant power of our existence."

It's Your Time to Heal

Patricia Bragg would not sugarcoat it. Creating and painting ageless health and beauty takes work, time, and focus. When *The Queen of Natural Living* sees anyone veering from Mother Nature's ways, she says, "We earn our health." However, building consistency takes time. Give yourself endless second chances to overcome past crippling habits. Embrace the power to heal, to leap, and to soar.

Patricia Bragg's legacy is her life—one of power, grace, humor, radiant health, and abundant joy. She exudes complete peace, yet not complacent. Beyond her wildest dreams, she is on fire with the mission of spreading health and ageless beauty. Now, unencumbered by the details of running a multimillion-dollar company, she is free to expand her creativity and vision. Her eyes sparkle with excitement for each new project. Our intention is that with the tools in this book you will smile and say, "I wouldn't trade the power and freedom of being my authentic self for anything."

This chapter of her life is her crowning glory. What do you want your legacy to be?

Action Steps

Patricia Bragg has always advocated meditation, deep breathing, and biofeedback to renew and replenish the nerves. She developed the "Constant Instant Practice," or "CIP," and says, "This is a process that rapidly reestablishes equilibrium in just a few moments and helps break the cycle of stress naturally at its source."

1. Constant Instant Practice (CIP)

Take five minutes to do these three simple steps anytime:

1. Sit in a comfortable position with a straight back and take a few deep cleansing breaths.
2. Consciously relax your muscles, starting at your feet and saying, "My feet are relaxed, my ankles are relaxed," etc. until you reach the top of your head.
3. Warm your hands by rubbing them vigorously and then immediately rub your hands over the front and back of each foot.

2. The Happiness Meditation

Janet Attwood and Chris Attwood write that: "The brain is very happy when you're focused on what you love. The more you focus on what you truly love and desire, the volume gets turned down in those parts of the limbic system where the destructive emotions of fear, anger, depression, and anxiety are controlled. This allows you to think more clearly.

You also turn up the volume in other parts of the limbic system that generate positive emotions. When this happens, you get a release of dopamine, endorphins, and a variety of stress-reducing hormones and neurotransmitters. The more you focus on what you love, the healthier you are likely to be, and the more you will feel the positive effects of those stress-reducing neurochemicals in your mind."

Happiness meditations can help you heal your limbic system as you grant permission for your inner healer, your Vital Force, to work and create a healthy and happy life—far beyond what your mind can imagine. Have you ever noticed how easy it is to grouse and complain, rather than to be joyful, even if things are going well? We tend to assign more attention to negative memories than positive ones.

With the happiness meditation, you're retraining your brain to value positive and happy memories over negative and painful ones, making joy your predominant state of mind. As you practice this meditation with all your senses engaged, you savor the memory as if it's happening again in present time. This literally changes the soft wiring of your brain.

Create a happiness meditation:

1. Prepare two stories to serve as meditations. Practice these five to ten minutes daily, for 21 days.
2. Start by writing a scene from your past. Choose one of the happiest moments of your life, when you felt healthy and life flowed effortlessly. Write about what you see, feel, smell, taste, and touch. Be specific. This is an example. I wrote about a time in Hawaii with my young children:

   I am sitting on a towel, under a big umbrella on my favorite beach. It's late afternoon and the sun is shining, but the heat of the day has passed, and a soft breeze touches my skin. The moment is perfect to soak up this heavenly place. I look out at the blue-green ocean and see my son, Luke, swimming with his best friend, Lino. They jump off a rock in the bay and cannonball into the water. I cheer them on, laughing and grinning from ear to ear, overflowing with joy. My daughter, Hana, is building a sandcastle next to me, and she's covering my feet in warm, soft sand. I look down at my body, which has birthed these two beautiful beings and feel overflowing love and acceptance. My skin is glowing and my eyes sparkle! I am strong, flexible, and healthy. I feel like I could do anything. A pulsing, radiant energy courses through my veins. I enjoy the most luscious tropical fruit salad, savoring every bite. The fragrance of pineapple and mango is like perfume in the air. I feel light and happy. Note: If you don't recall a day when you felt safe and healthy, invent one. Your life starts **now**.

3. Next, write another story about a future moment when you are happy, healthy, and life is flowing. Write from your heart about what you'd like to see in front of you. Are you at a dream job? Are you in the creative dream world of painting a picture? Are you looking your beloved in the eye—feeling your love reciprocated? Are you cozy in the living room of your new home? Are you on fire from the passion for a new business?

4. In a journal, write a happiness meditation memory.

5. Then, write your future self happiness meditation. This is an example of my future self meditation:

As I stand in my backyard on a late September day, the garden is bursting with goodness! I see rows of lettuce, carrots, beets, and zucchini so thick that the dark, rich mulch from which they come is almost completely hidden. I did this! I created the garden that feeds our family. This is a satisfaction I had never experienced. I feel so grateful for these strong arms that carried the compost, dug in the dirt, wielded a big shovel as if I were 20 years old. My legs are tan and muscular and my back unflinching as I carry another big bag of fertilizer to the back of the yard. My energy is unstoppable. I am so happy here, so filled with peace and joy. The birds serenade me as I scoop my hands into the cool, dark ground, smiling at the fat worms whose wriggly squirms aerate the dirt, making this possible. I smell the lavender and rosemary from the herb garden and taste a sweet snap pea that is crawling up the trellis. Delicious! I could stay here all day. I am totally fulfilled. Life is so good.

3. Happiness Meditation Affirmations

When you finish writing your happiness and future self meditations, write a few sentences which sum up the feelings of your meditations. Stand up and say these aloud a few times, without hesitation and with great confidence. You claim your birthright. When you claim strength, joy, and love, another person's joy is undiminished. The more we claim our birthright of health and happiness, the greater our capacity to embody all that is possible. When I was healing, meeting people who recovered their health gave me courage. Our greatest legacy is to establish our lives as happy, full, and as well lived as possible. This is how we honor those who came before us, and those who will come after us.

Every day, morning and night, look into a mirror and confidently say your affirmations aloud. Find a comfortable and quiet space in your house to read your stories. Start by taking slow, deep breaths, exhaling the limitations you were taught. Then, breathe in the incredible possibilities ahead of you.

4. Creating Motivation

Make a list of what outcomes might inspire you:

- Less pain
- Feeling joy
- Greater energy
- To paint, write, and dance
- To love who I see in the mirror
- To feel pleasure and sensuality
- The confidence to change careers
- To run and play with my dear ones
- The courage to put on a bathing suit

What are your motivators?

In Conclusion

We claim our power when we face our demons, put ourselves first, and refuse to accept society's definition of our worth as well as what or who defines beauty.

This means becoming free. To do that, we must resuscitate our nervous systems, heal our bodies, and rediscover our own beauty. That frees us and leads us, unfailingly, to authentic power. Feminine power. The kind of power with no time for self-sabotage—she's too busy having fun, planting flowers, wearing sparkles, and charming steak-lovers into loving fresh salads.

Yes, that's Patricia Bragg's style of power, which comes from her living her truth. To love our bodies, see our beauty, and reclaim our power is a lifelong journey. Together, through the wisdom of Mother Nature's teachings and Patricia Bragg's mentorship, you will learn to liberate yourself from the mind and body toxins that bind, and open to the unchained happiness that is your birthright.

Revolutionary Beauty Cynthia James

Cynthia James is an international speaker, best-selling author, and life coach.

Cynthia: *I always found myself comparing my face and body to others. As an African American, I vacillated between comparing myself to Caucasian standards for beauty and the color system in my own community. For some, I was too light to be considered Black. For others, my hair was too nappy to be considered beautiful.*

When I was in junior high, we were required to take swimming and it bought out terror in the Black girls! We wore swim caps, but the dread of having our hair get wet and be embarrassed with nappy hair was the topic of many conversations. One day, my swim cap came off in the pool and I was devastated. I put a scarf on my head and asked the teacher if I could go home for an hour. I shared how embarrassing it was to have others make fun of my hair, but she would not budge. So, I went anyway. I got in trouble and my mother had to come to school and explain to the principal and the teacher the vulnerable state caused within me. They had no interest in listening to her. So, going forward, my mother straightened my hair with hot combs and lye based products. It was often painful and I found it excruciating.

In my early thirties, I discovered that my significant other was cheating on me. It was humbling. Each time I would take him back after a promise never to do it again. I found a therapist and was completely dedicated to healing my lack of self-love. That was monumental to me! My therapist was very kind, and he witnessed me eating 3 Musketeers bars when I was stressed, or close to a breakthrough. He gently invited me to look at my inner rage, and I learned that the chocolate and sugar were distractions. When he asked me to release some of that anger, consciously, I resisted. Finally, after me coming and leaving a few times, we got to the deep sadness and wounds that had held me hostage most of my life. He invited me to walk every day, to get the energy out of my body, and to begin to connect with my feelings.

It was during this time that I was also engaged in a spiritual community that encouraged me to journal and connect to our spiritual being. Then, I enrolled in a self-defense course. The women were taught to fight off men in various situations and I cried through the entire graduation. The outcome was miraculous. I found my voice. I found inner strength. I felt so empowered and strong. That moment was a true turning point. I entered a Master's Program in Spiritual Psychology and became a leadership coach for women. Today, my coaching work is focused on the mind-body connection. I teach clients to learn to listen to the body's language.

I am 71 and feel that being my age is a great gift. I am fearless and daring. I have learned to love myself. I have learned to trust my intuitive knowing and only share my life with people that complement my values. My health is non-negotiable. I have learned that your commitment to your body and your health is imperative!

MODULE 2

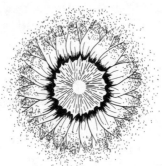

Episode 4
LET'S BEGIN AT THE
BEGINNING: PURIFICATION

"Age is a number and mine is unlisted."
—Patricia Bragg, Health Pioneer and Author

Why Purify?

Purification is the key component to Revolutionary Beauty. Due to the toxicity of our planet—plus modern-day stress—internal cleansing is more important than most medical practitioners realize. Surprisingly, few dermatologists are aware of the relationship between purification and beautiful skin.

Revolutionary Beauty is all about creating timeless beauty from within. The source of glowing skin is vibrant health. However, nutritious food and high quality supplements are not enough to achieve radical health in our current environment. Our organs are overwhelmed with toxins! The goal of purification is to gently facilitate the release of poisons. The exciting news is that you can do the purification practices outlined in this module in the privacy of your home. You will become captain of your ship, and goddess of your spa!

The skin is the largest organ of the body, a critical channel of detoxification. Toxic overload is the source of breakouts, acne, cellulite, wrinkles, and eczema. If we do not purify the body, we cannot assimilate vital nutrients. Neurotoxins affect our mood and ability to feel joy and excitement.

Do you feel utterly hopeless at times?

Or, do you feel *blah*, as if nothing really matters? I've heard that confession from thousands of clients—what a terrifying admission. They call themselves *weak* and *lazy*, but they are not! The source of crippling fatigue and brain fog is toxicity.

The value of purification has been recognized for thousands of years. Until this century, the practice of purification was not a fundamental facet of daily life. In fact, the focus on cleanliness, in general, is relatively new to human beings. Handwashing has only been practiced for the last two hundred years. This simple practice was generally enough to protect the immune health of our great-grandparents and served them well. They were allowed to literally get their hands dirty—and then wash off the dirt.

Triple board-certified physician and scientist Dr. Zach Bush says that today, immunity is compromised because the gut microbiome is 90 percent less diverse than in previous generations. What was the source of that diverse microbiome? Soil. Our ancestors benefited from a closer relationship with mother earth, plus a more diverse gut microbiome. They spent their days with hands in the dirt, foraging or growing food. Children played freely outside. Many people lived predominantly outdoors. Bacteria isn't all bad.

In the last century, environmental toxins have changed that for us. Mother earth is bombarded with chemicals, and so are we. Two billion pounds of contaminants are poured into American soil each year. We connect with as many as 2,500 chemicals daily, through the air, water, and food.

Paul Bragg spoke about the link between toxins and disease nearly 100 years ago. In the late 1940s, he penned an entire series of books on the subject. Bragg convinced his friend Rachel Carlson to write *Silent Spring* in 1966. This ground-breaking best seller was the first mainstream publication to alert Americans of chemical dangers in food, air, and water. At that time, the public was unaware of the consequences of those poisons. In the 1960s, I was the only child in my school who carried an inhaler in her lunchbox. Today, one of four kids suffers from asthma.

The statistics are staggering. The World Health Organization reports that one of three Americans is obese. Three of five between 25-40 struggle with infertility. One of four is depressed. Their studies project that in the next decade, one in eight children will be diagnosed with some form of autism. One of two adults will fight cancer and diabetes. Given these numbers, why is feeling and looking beautiful so important? Why are billions spent yearly on skincare products and make-up? Health care professionals scratch their heads about this reality. Beauty matters for a reason. Our DNA prioritizes beauty. We are hardwired to exalt beauty. Beauty is where life begins, which feeds our soul. When you gaze at your beloved or your child's face, what do you say? How beautiful they are.

All drugs—even ones that save lives—deliver toxic side effects that linger in our bodies until we purify them. It is a myth that the body releases these toxins through breathing and elimination. If that were true, autoimmune disease, digestive issues, and depression would not be some of our nation's most pressing health care concerns. Instead, gastroenterologists treat millions of bloated, unhappy bellies daily. Antacids and laxatives are top selling over-the-counter medications. Picture pouring a 25-pound sack of cement into a full dumpster. That is the state of many colons I have seen as a colon hydrotherapist. A medical colleague of mine disputed that fact until he came into my office for his first treatment!

Modern medicine is a gift in certain situations. Who isn't grateful for pain relievers after surgery? Unfortunately, they are often overprescribed. Residual toxins are not eliminated by exercise, because they are deeply embedded in the body's tissues and cells. In addiction cases, accumulated toxins are not eliminated by entering a rehab facility. That is not the goal of most rehab programs. The focus is to kick the addiction. You are on your own when it comes to purifying and restoring your organs.

The side effects of pharmaceuticals, such as anesthesia, antibiotics, statins, and pain-killers may last years if untreated. Symptoms from this toxic burden include depression, anxiety, sleep issues, extreme fatigue, digestive stress, loss of libido, hormone imbalance, adrenal collapse, weight gain, immune system breakdown, neuralgia, and neuropathy. Any one of these rob us of our vitality, right before our eyes. This is why purification is so critical. We predict that in the next decade, Revolutionary Beauty's innovative, unconventional secrets to agelessness will be as common as washing your hands.

Youth is not lost on the young. Sparkle, delight, and open-hearted optimism can be reclaimed and nurtured at any age. Like Patricia Bragg, the Revolutionary Beauties you will meet in this book are happier and healthier than they have ever been. They smile at their reflection and embrace each new tomorrow. We can, and will have a strong immune system, an exuberant attitude, and taut, glowing, cellulite-free skin. Though the purification practices in this episode are simple, the greater challenge may be walking away from your to-do list. As women, we are conditioned to take care of everyone else first. Revolutionary Beauties treat themselves like queens because they know their worth. If burnout, stress, and toxicity have cast a shadow on your crown, now is your moment to step from darkness into the sunlight.

Lymphatic Health: River of Life

Not to be confused with the limbic system in the brain, the lymphatic system is the fluid that flows between tissues and organs. This fluid carries important disease fighting white blood cells and flushes toxins and waste. If the study of the lymphatic system is new to you, you are not alone. Called the *river of life*, lymphatic fluid comprises much of the 75 percent of water in our bodies. In charge of our flow of energy, rate of metabolism, and stamina, the lymphatic system also manages our level of inflammation. This is a weighty and impressive responsibility, as the American Medical Association (AMA) has recognized inflammation as the source of all diseases.

We experience inflammation as the swelling under our jaw when we have a cold, and puffiness in the morning when our ankles appear to have doubled in size. Inflammation is the source of chronic pain. That frustrating *tire around the middle*, as well as tummy bloat, is the result of inflammation. Body inflammation is calculated according to genetics, plus the degree of toxicity, stress, and lifestyle choices. In this episode, we target the latter three, which we can control.

Stress and the Inflammation Lifestyle

The lymphatic fluid, called *interstitial fluid*, runs from head to toe. There is a continuous interchange between the body's trillion cells and interstitial fluid, which is grayish in color. Pressure from the arteries moves this fluid from the cells, creating continuous circulation. As toxins are picked up by tiny lymphatic tubes or ducts, they are sent through the lymph vessels to be cleansed. The cells are constantly bathed, flushed, hydrated, oxygenated, fed, and massaged.

If toxins are not carried away, the living cells become compromised and die. When lymph fluid is healthy, it flows like a wave, with a watery consistency. But when the lymph is inflamed, the consistency is thick like glue. This is what creates cellulite, which is the deposit of toxic waste in fatty tissues.

What you need to know about the lymphatic system is that unlike the blood system—which is pumped by the heart—the lymphatic system has no pump. The lymphatic system depends upon the contraction of muscles to move the fluid. Two other modalities that flush the lymphatic system are dry skin brushing and jumping on a rebounder.

At certain phases along the lymphatic channels, lymph nodes collect toxins from disease producing bacteria and cancerous growths. Yes, you read the words "cancerous growths." According to immunologist Lawrence Burton, PhD, cancer and infection are always present in our bodies. Regardless, natural immunity prevents us from actually developing disease. In other words, we all carry cancer cells within our bodies, but our lymph nodes prevent the spread of disease by keeping these cancer cells localized. A healthy immune system also successfully battles infection. You can see why the lymphatic system is so important! This invaluable cleansing fluid literally saves our lives daily.

I worked as a colon therapist and gut health specialist for two decades before I understood the value of lymphatic therapy. I had received a few lymphatic drainage sessions over the years, with no dramatic results. Then, I met a true master, Allen Mills, founder of the Center for Lymphatic Health in Santa Barbara. Lymphatic drainage therapy is a massage using gentle, intentional movements that unstick the bond between protein molecules in the lymph nodes to get the lymphatic fluid moving again. Allen was a firm believer in the link between lymphatic and colon health. I witnessed miracles in the clients that he referred to me. Yet, it took my own health crisis for me to experience the power of lymphatic drainage.

Stress Goes to Breasts

At my visit with my nurse practitioner for my PAP smear, she said, "Julia, you have cysts that I didn't feel last year. I know there's no history of breast cancer in your family, but I'm concerned. I'm sure it's nothing, but we're going to keep an eye on this. I want to see you in three months. Don't worry. It's probably hormones or stress."

"Don't worry" are two of the most stress producing words in the English language. I immediately called Allen and made an appointment. For my first lymphatic session, he checked the lymph nodes in my body. Allen had a knack for making patients feel safe. Once he checked key lymphatic areas for suspect spots, he began to massage those stuck places with subtle movements until smooth. He also lightly touched my skin with the light filled wands of a machine called a Lymph Star. This machine amplifies the body's ability to separate the bond between the protein molecules, unclogging lymphatic nodes and ducts.

"I feel congestion in your breasts," he said. "And in your lungs and your uterus—in fact, everywhere!" I was amazed at his sensitivity. Allen told me two-thirds of our lymph is palpable and can be felt and seen right beneath the surface of the skin. "We can handle this," he said calmly, which relaxed me.

Lymphatic Health: Key to Vitality and Purification

I dry brushed my skin each morning and received a series of 12 lymphatic massages. In six months, the cysts were healed.

As important as a positive mindset is, this is not all magical thinking. Dr. Arthur Guyton, Professor and Chairman of the Department of Physiology and Biophysics at the University of Mississippi School of Medicine did studies that show us a sluggish lymphatic system can not only cause cysts, but also encourage diseases such as cancer, heart attacks, strokes, diabetes, kidney failure, and chronic problems like headaches, depression, anxiety, and allergies. A sluggish lymphatic system is usually the reason you catch every cold and flu that comes along. Varicose veins, hemorrhoids, and blood clots can also be a result of this condition.

Have you ever looked in the mirror, and seemed so swollen you wished you could pop yourself like a balloon? The root cause is often a sluggish lymphatic system. And, like all parts of the body, the lymph is entirely capable of healing.

In many European countries, prescribing lymphatic drainage therapy is a doctor's first course of action. They find that many issues resolve after a series of treatments and further intervention is not necessary. In America, lymphatic drainage therapy has not yet been welcomed into mainstream medicine. However, this modality is breaking ground as a key to safeguard women's breast health.

It's Swell Not to be Swollen

You can feel swollen lymph nodes below your ears, below your collarbone, under your armpits into your breast (men, too), and in the crease between the thigh and the pelvic area, as well as under your jaw. You might feel some small bumps or lumps when you touch these areas, or grittiness from the swelling of water retention, called *edema*. All these lumps and bumps are signs of blocked lymphatic nodes and vessels.

In western medicine, clogged lymph nodes are often removed. Healing the lymph is a far better long-term solution to the problem of inflammation, congestion, and disease.

If you have wrestled with a weight loss program for years to no avail, you may be amazed at the inches that melt off after implementing the lymph healing rituals in this book, especially if you pair them with "CARE Colon Cleansing." All women are busy, so most of these rituals take less than ten minutes a day. Because everyone needs one rejuvenation day a week, we encourage you to set aside a few hours regularly for the longer rituals. These will become your most treasured moments. Self-care is not selfish—it is sacred.

Lymphatic drainage allows our lymphatic system to heal, reduces swelling, fine lines, and our susceptibility to more serious issues. This process is safe and easy for anyone to do. Lymphatic drainage allows the lymph to drain without stimulating blood flow the way ultrasound does. Gentle, light movements unstick the bond between the protein molecules and get the lymphatic fluid moving.

Two years later, I was rear-ended in my car. I sustained whiplash and a concussion. Two months later, the cysts returned. We have a saying in my clinic, "Stress goes to our breasts."

I did another series with Allen and continued my dry skin brushing, and the cysts again disappeared! Allen's absolute faith in the body's ability to heal reminded me of the healing powers within ourselves, and of someone whose teachings had saved me years before—Patricia Bragg.

Patricia has been recommending and practicing dry skin brushing for years. When I reached my own *aha moment* as to the significance of lymphatic health—which took a personal experience—my curiosity was piqued as to why this modality had been so neglected. Yet, two of the most supportive and beneficial therapies to improve lymphatic health are simple and easy: dry-skin brushing and lymphatic drainage massage.

Action Steps

CARE Rituals to Heal the Lymph

Lymphatic massage is safe, easy, and enjoyable—especially by trained professionals. But anyone can do two other easy practices at home to pump and purify the lymphatic system. The first is dry skin brushing, which will instantly give you more energy and reduce swelling with the added benefit of saying "bye-bye" to the cottage cheese we call cellulite. The second home therapy for healing the lymph is rebounding on a small trampoline.

1. How to Dry Brush Your Skin

First, you'll need a high quality dry brush. Look for one with bristles made from natural materials that are stiff, but still soft when you brush your skin. Choose a brush with a long handle so that you can reach your entire back and other hard to reach spots. Dry skin brushing should be done daily for optimal results, or even twice a day if you like. Always brush toward your heart, which is best for circulation and the lymphatic system. You can brush your entire body, including your feet. See the chart below for how to skin brush, and follow these guidelines.

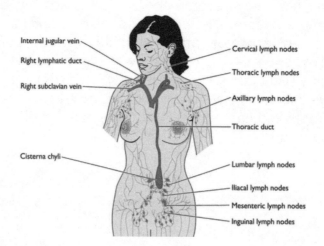

Start at your belly and work in circles counterclockwise. Then, brush from your belly upwards to your heart. Next, brush your arms, neck, and chest. The stimulation on your upper chest, just below your throat, to your thymus gland, is effective to energize your immune system. Now, work your way up your legs and make sure to do the insides of your thighs, where many lymph nodes are located. Brush your neck and bottom. Avoid brushing your face, your genitals, or any areas with rashes or abrasions, including varicose veins. Notice how soft your skin feels after you brush. The pressure you apply while while brushing your skin should be firm, but not painful (avoid scrubbing). Your skin may be a little pink after your first session (not red or irritated). An average dry skin brushing session may last between two and 20 minutes.

If you experience issues with inflammation or are injured, skin brushing helps to reduce swelling. Park yourself with your brush in front of your favorite TV show or film, or listen to music, and brush for 30-45 minutes. You will be amazed how good you will feel, and how dramatically puffiness diminishes.

To experience lymphatic drainage therapy, contact a well trained practitioner and register for a session, or series. For optimal results, know that you are giving yourself one of the most powerful healing techniques that exist. Ask the practitioner to show you places on your body where you're most congested, so you can work on them in between sessions.

2. Jumping for Joy

If you struggle with depression or feeling *blah*, as if you have no gas in the tank, precede your happiness meditation from the previous episode with five to eight minutes of bouncing on a rebounder or trampoline, or even on your bed if you don't mind giving your mattress a workout!

Bouncing moves the lymph and pumps endorphins—also good for building core muscles. Try ten minutes a day, and watch your booty lift and your tummy flatten—what better way to lift your spirits! Doing this practice daily can be a game changer if you deal with anxiety or depression. Bouncing is fun and the best mood changer in the world. You need not jump high, especially if balance is a challenge. Simply bounce gently to your favorite music.

My Family's Bouncing Story

When my kids and I were going through a difficult time during my divorce (they were six and eleven), each of us experienced conflicted and confused feelings on a daily basis. Jumping on the trampoline became a daily routine for all of us—the ten minutes before breakfast. Sometimes when we marched outside, we started out quiet and solemn. Yet, within five minutes we were laughing. The kids were smiling again and feeling like themselves, letting go of the stress of the situation that didn't belong to them. They got to be kids again, kids without the weight of this transition on their shoulders.

At night, we repeated our jumping, followed by a happiness meditation or prayers that we would make up in that moment. We all spoke from our hearts with no feelings censored. We ended with a meditation of memories to make us happy.

Bouncing on the trampoline activated our lymphatic systems, boosted our endorphins in a matter of minutes, and brought joy. The Happiness Meditation gave us peace and connection. Both activities prepared us for the important work of the subconscious.

3. The Seven-Day Trial

Do both of these—bouncing and dry-brushing—daily for seven days, particularly before performing your own happiness meditation and affirmations. This is a recipe for clarity and calm, especially during times of transition, crisis, and change. You will be amazed at how much better you will feel. And once you feel better, your seven-day trial will easily turn into a weekly, if not daily habit. Excellent rebounders with safe springs are available online.

In Conclusion

Lymphatic drainage—including dry brushing, rebounding, and massage—allows the lymph nodes to drain without stimulating blood flow the way ultrasound does. While ultrasound therapy can help promote healing of a sore muscle or bruise, normally this is not done at home. Dry skin brushing, rebounding, and meditating help to calm the mind and body, detoxify our lymphatic system, and cleanse from the inside out—which is the goal of Revolutionary Beauty.

Conditions improved by lymphatic therapy:

- Cellulite
- Chronic pain
- Chronic fatigue
- Prostate issues
- Allergies and asthma
- Regulation of periods
- Swollen hands and feet
- Headaches and migraines
- Breast congestion and cysts
- Bloating and digestive issues such as IBS or colitis
- Arthritis or any condition caused by inflammation

Revolutionary Beauty Mae West

You may know Mae West as the sultry screen star, controversial playwright, singer, and author whose career spanned seven decades. In 1935, she was the second highest paid person in the United States behind publisher William Randolph Hearst.

What the public did not know is that Ms. West was a Revolutionary Beauty who practiced every ritual outlined in this book, from an organic diet to colon cleansing, meditation, exercise, and plenty of time in bed (some of it sleeping). Enjoy these excerpts from her autobiography, *Sex, Health, and ESP*.

Mae: *Whenever I give an interview, someone says, "Miss West, you look fabulous! How do you do it?" As always, I get right to the point! "Positive thinking and no drinkin!"*

Goodness may have had nothing to do with my diamonds, but it has everything to do with my health. I believe that if you don't take care of yourself, nobody else will. And so, all my life, I've taken every measure to pamper and protect myself.

My face is free of lines and wrinkles, and I have never had any kind of facelift or plastic surgery. My looks don't come from good fortune—or from any fortune spent on cosmetics. They are a result of a lifetime of good health habits, and those habits can work for anyone.

The time to begin taking care of yourself isn't when it becomes necessary—it's way before. I have always had to be in top physical form to meet the demands of my work. I've gotten my rest every night—or part of every night, anyway! I've never smoked, and the only time I've held a cigarette has been when it was part of characterization. Even then I had somebody else light it for me. And I've never liked liquor! A guy has plenty to look at when he comes up to see me, but he won't see a bottle or an ashtray!

Long before recent cholesterol studies were made, I developed the right eating habits. Natural foods, and naturally healthy foods, have always been on my table.

When I go to a party, I often arrive after dinner, knowing it's better for my health. I've always been the kind of girl who not only gets second looks but gives them; and so, when I sit down to a meal at somebody's house, I eat only what I would eat in my own home, not foods I wouldn't ordinarily consume.

I've never had to go on a major diet, but there have been times—such as after the holidays—when I find that I picked up some extra weight. A girl should handle excess pounds like she would guys—drop 'em fast!

I stay away from fried foods; don't drink coffee and only eat unsweetened chocolate. I drink several glasses of water a day, but never from the tap. Spring water or mineral water is far more healthful.

For breakfast, like so many of the good things in life, I have this meal in bed. A single slice of toasted whole grain bread (no GMO's in Mae's time) with one egg and weak tea with no sugar. For lunch, I have organically grown fruit, and for dinner, clean, freshly prepared chicken broth or a green salad, and then either chicken, steak, or fish. I always eat a green vegetable at dinner, sometimes a baked potato or brown rice, and use sea salt in light amounts. For dessert, I'll have fruit. That's the Mae West plan for good eating!

I also get plenty of exercise. I'm happy, too, with the people around me. Stay away from anything and anyone unpleasant; that's my motto, and I live by it.

Clean Livin'

Now I'll pass along an important health secret of mine, perhaps the most important of all. It concerns cleanliness, the interior kind. Just as our faces and bodies must be kept clean and free of dirt, our insides need constant cleansing. Our colons can become lined with unwanted substances and distorted out of shape. The result of this neglect shows itself in what we call the signs of old age: dull skin, big stomachs, and numerous health disorders. I started this colon cleansing habit in 1928!

Putrid matter is poisonous and too many people walk around loaded with poison. Indigestion, poor skin, even cancer, these can be caused by poisons in our body. By cleaning our system, we can rid ourselves of potential dangers before they have a chance to harm us.

The importance of removing every trace of putrid matter from the body can't be stressed enough.

Now you know my secrets for good health!

MODULE 2

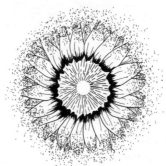

Episode 5
HAPPY GUT, HAPPY LIFE:
BEAUTY BEGINS IN THE COLON

"You are never too old to become younger!"

—Mae West, Film Star, Playwright, Singer and Author

I don't know how people detoxify effectively without colon cleansing. Actually, I do know. They suffer unnecessarily. Colon cleansing—whether done at home or by professional colon hydrotherapists—drastically reduces uncomfortable symptoms of toxicity. These include headaches, anxiety, insomnia, gas, bloating, flu-like symptoms, fatigue, and even depression.

In my twenties, while living on the east coast, I came to New York City to receive colonics from an elegant woman in her late eighties. Her exquisite office was on Fifth Avenue off Central Park. She regaled me with stories of giving colonics to the silent film stars of the 1930s and 1940s. These well-known beauties would have been called *health nuts* in their day. Many were followers of pioneer authors Paul Bragg and Dr. Henry Bieler (*Food is Your Best Medicine*). Theirs were the first books written to promote a healthy diet as an antidote for disease, as well as for antiaging. Gloria Swanson and Greta Garbo were two of their famous proteges.

Botox had not yet been invented to smooth the furrowed brows of these Hollywood beauties. They needed to find another way. *The Gut Health Goddess of Fifth Avenue* shared that Mae West credited coffee colonics for her flawless skin and youthful glow. Leave it to a woman like Mae West, ahead of her time in many ways, to discover one of the best-kept secrets of natural beauty. Mae stated, "I believe in censorship; I've made a fortune out of it."

It may not have been *in vogue* for *turn of the century women* to speak candidly about beauty rituals. Lucky for us, times have changed. The 2020 "Beautiful People Issue" of *People Magazine* featured Revolutionary Beauties Goldie Hawn and Kate Hudson on the cover. The ageless mother-daughter duo shared their beauty secrets:

Goldie: *The best beauty advice that I passed down to my daughter is ...*

Kate: *Green juice.*

Goldie: *Yes, and get your sleep, clear your mind. Meditate.*

Kate: *Saunas. Colonics. (Laughs)*

Goldie: *Oh yeah. Why wasn't that #1? (Laughs)*

When I began my serious detoxification program, two decades of pharmaceutical drugs were stored in my young body. Twice, during fasts and cleanses, my body was covered with boils for thirty days straight. I couldn't concentrate to save my life, and the migraines lasted for weeks. After I began colon cleansing, my skin cleared, the migraines stopped. The asthma completely abated. The colitis healed.

My tummy flattened, without gas or bloating. Yet, above all, the return of my sense of peace and profound joy was as significant as the ability to breathe without a wheeze.

Over the last forty years, I have witnessed my clients experience a similar transformation. Whether their original intention for receiving colonics was to heal allergies or irritable bowel syndrome, nearly all report an elevated mood and lightness of being.

Happy Gut, Happy Life

If the belly is happy, we're happy! That is because 90 percent of serotonin, the neurotransmitter that creates happiness, is synthesized in the gut. In 1998, New York City's Columbia University's College of Physicians and Surgeons Professor Dr. Michael Gershon, MD, wrote a groundbreaking book, *The Second Brain*. This research represented a quantum leap in medical knowledge. The connection between the gut and the brain, as newly described by science, was an epiphany. The key connector is the vagus nerve. This giant highway carries transmissions to and from the gut and the brain.

In fact, the vagus nerve carries more information from the gut to the brain than from the brain to the gut. This is why the term *second brain* is so relevant. Science validated the connections between mental health, gut health, and the microbiome, a collection of bacteria that live in the gut. Think of your microbiome—also called intestinal flora—as a treasure chest whose booty represents vitality, happiness, and immune health. A healthy colon is both the map and the key to that treasure chest!

The question people are most reticent to ask is, "Is colon hydrotherapy painful?" Surprisingly, this procedure is comfortable and relaxing. Clients often describe feeling euphoric following a session. With the release of toxins, the nervous system does a happy dance! The boost of serotonin is palpable. Because the gut and the brain are connected, colon therapy is an excellent modality to heal emotional trauma and limbic brain injuries. The release of toxins brings awareness to physical and emotional areas that have remained in the dark for years. Memories are held in the cells. To release that trauma is the beginning of a new life. The colon is a center of release for early sexual abuse and PTSD. I have worked with many survivors whose long-standing physical and emotional issues shifted during their treatments.

Anatomy of the Colon

Most colons are in trouble. The colon, also called the large intestine, is the last six feet of the digestive tract. This organ is located at the end of the small intestine. When the colon lacks muscle tone, constipation is a given. Did you know that bad breath can originate from waste in your colon? That is why those mints don't always work. An apt phrase that I learned years ago is, "Machinery rusts and people rot!"

The colon can expand with waste to touch every major organ in the human body except the brain. Each of these organs may be compressed and crushed by a clogged colon: the lungs, liver, gallbladder, pancreas, kidneys, adrenals, uterus, and prostate. Constipation creates an infinite variety of health problems.

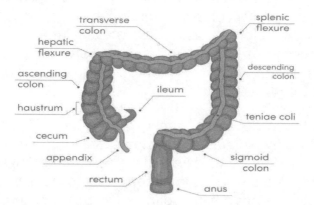

The colon is lined with pockets from beginning to end with bulbous pouches that contract similarly to how a snake moves. Trouble begins when fecal debris is stuck in these areas. When worms and parasites hide out in these pockets and pouches, headaches, nausea, and depression can occur. When John Wayne donated his body to science, forty pounds of toxic waste was hiding in his colon. But the trophy goes to Elvis. At the time of his death, fifty pounds of waste was uncovered in his!

With wavelike motions called peristalsis, the colon moves waste from the cecum through the rectum. Found near the ileac valve, below the right hip is a small, worm-like sack about three inches long. This is known as the appendix. The appendix is a lymphatic organ whose primary job is to keep the ileocecal valve free of infection and inflammation. We know what happens when this organ is toxic—appendicitis!

If colonic waste has putrefied and fermented, the bloodstream becomes polluted. The liquid that would otherwise be used by the body as nutrition becomes toxemia. This toxemia slows the metabolism to a mere gasp. Without a strong metabolism, a low calorie diet plus high-powered exercise fails to result in weight loss.

All food must pass through twenty-two feet of the small intestine to reach the colon. The Standard American diet—white bread, processed meat, and fake fat—is so gluey and toxic that these foods are not assimilated or eliminated rapidly. Few people can brag about a bowel movement after each meal. If small children live with you, look in the toilet after they go. The amount of poop you will see resembles a Great Dane's! That is a healthy functioning colon.

Do you know that low back pain may be the result of bowel distress? As a former back pain sufferer, when I discovered colon cleansing and food combining, the pain disappeared. I advocate for gentle spinal manipulations and chiropractors.

Yet, no manipulation accomplishes what colon cleansing does for chronic back pain from gas and undigested food.

Why Metabolism Grinds to a Halt

Dr. Michael Galitzer, nationally recognized longevity expert, writes in his book, *Outstanding Health*:

"The surface area of the intestines is more than 200 square yards. Within that expanse, it is all too common that an accumulation of impacted feces, waste, toxins, and other matter can occur. Thus, even though you may be having at least one daily bowel moment (two per day is ideal), your colon may not be healthy. The buildup of waste matter along the colon tract can result in a wide array of health problems, including diminished absorption of nutrients, suppressed immune function, inflammation, leaky gut syndrome, and other gastrointestinal problems. This is why I often recommend that my patients consider having a few colon hydrotherapy sessions."

When the blood is overburdened with toxic waste, the liver picks up the slack. Next comes the bladder, sitting in front of the last part of the intestine. When toxins leak into the bladder, inflammation, infection, and chronic discomfort follow. *Talk about leaking.* Adult diapers are a billion dollar industry!

At this point, the toxic burden is dumped into the lymphatic system. This is why lymphatic drainage is an integral part of detoxification. Master lymphatic therapist Allen Mills occasionally refused to see a client who was presenting signs of toxemia—headaches, edema, body aches—until they did some form of colon cleansing.

Famous health spas such as Hippocrates Health in Palm Beach, Florida and We Care in Palm Desert, California offer professional colonics. These are particularly effective to assist fasting clients in doing longer cleanses. Colon cleansing is a safe and effective method of releasing toxins. By stimulating the production of the gut's serotonin, colon cleansing creates a sense of deep peace—that *all is right with the world* feeling. However, a visit to a spa is not required to regenerate your health, and enjoy this buoyancy. You can practice colon cleansing at home safely and effectively.

CARE Colon Cleansing

I am often asked the question, "Can a person do too much colon cleansing?" The answer is "yes." The tendency to think *more is better* is a misguided one. For example, as a student at Hippocrates Health Institute, while participating in a fruit and vegetable cleanse, one guest consumed forty oranges in one day. Full recovery from the effects of its high sugar content and acidity took two weeks! However, gentle colon cleansing done seasonally—or even weekly or monthly—is safe.

While the body flushes toxins during colon cleansing, electrolytes are also lost. Add sugar-free electrolytes to your drinking water after a home enema or colonic to rebalance the body. As for probiotics, a healthy body restores gut flora within twenty-four hours of colon cleansing. Yet, probiotic supplementation is always worthwhile, since many people's bodies do not manufacture a sufficient amount.

The power of colon cleansing is not merely in emptying the impacted waste from the colon. This practice is key to detoxifying the liver and releasing toxins that irritate the nervous system. Liver and gallbladder cleanses have become popular in the last 20 years, and for good reason. The liver works overtime to flush toxins of processed foods, fake fats, pesticides, and environmental poisons. Colon cleansing of some kind is always recommended after these flushes—for optimal results—before as well. The liver can only release toxins if the colon is empty. Otherwise, the poison is recirculated.

This results in toxins being released directly into the blood-stream, which defeats the purpose of the flush. If you do a liver or gallbladder flush, follow with a colon cleanse.

I have seen dozens of clients become extremely ill after liver flushes. At the time, they believed the issue was a *detoxification reaction* originating from the idea that "you get worse before you get better." Although sometimes true, in this case, these symptoms are avoidable. Illness after any health practice is a red flag to seek professional guidance.

For answers to your specific questions, consult a detoxification expert or professional colon therapist (see Resource Guide). As my own guinea pig for dozens of health related experiments, I know this only too well.

Colon cleansing reduces inflammation and chronic pain. This practice may also boost energy, lift spirits, and revitalize your skin. Although professional treatment sessions are wonderful luxuries, you can purify and transform on your own. Colon therapy is truly the best-kept secret of joy, vitality, and ageless beauty. No doctor can inject radiance into our faces. We have to do that ourselves. And, we can!

Action Steps

Colon Cleansing 101

Three ways to cleanse the colon are as follows:

1. Herbal and saltwater ingestible cleanses
2. Do-it-yourself at home enemas
3. Professional colonics

1. Herbal and Saltwater Ingestible Cleanses

Herbal Cleanses—These involve ingesting herbal formulas that sweep through your colon to remove waste.

You do not want to use a laxative, or any product containing inflammatory herbs such as senna or cascara sagrada. After searching for a safe, gentle, and effective formula for my clients, I created the detoxifying Happy Gut Cleanse. Even those who never experience constipation appreciate extra help while traveling.

Laxatives work by irritating the colon, which causes inflammation—exactly what we are trying to avoid. If used regularly, laxatives can prevent the colon from working. I have seen hundreds of laxative dependent clients over the years, from ages 18 to 98. If you struggle with constipation, the prescription for healing includes staying well hydrated, using a gentle herbal detoxification formula, and embarking on a series of the colon cleanse practices outlined below (plus the health practices outlined in this book). In my experience, constipation is not always relieved just by adding more fiber to the diet. In fact, if diagnosed with IBS or colitis; gas or bloating, the condition may be worsened by using fiber. The key is cleansing the colon and stimulating peristalsis so that it naturally begins working again.

Flaxseed Infusion—Paul Bragg spoke and wrote about the health benefits of flaxseeds over one hundred years ago. They are a rich source of Omega-3 fatty acids. They help repair cells and tissues, transport oxygen, satisfy hunger, and increase metabolic rates. Bragg recommended making flaxseeds into a tea as a gentle cleanse for the digestive system. Below is Paul Bragg's original recipe for a flaxseed tea, which as an infusion does not introduce fiber into the intestines, so it is a great choice for sensitive stomachs—gentle, yet effective.

Boil 8 ounces of water with 2 teaspoons flaxseeds for 2-3 minutes. Steep for another 3-4 minutes. Then, strain while hot, and drink. The gelatinous quality of the flaxseeds, as well as many of the nutrients, will be retained in the water.

If you want additional fiber, you may drink the seeds as well. This infusion can be used regularly to stimulate healthy peristalsis and eliminate toxins.

Saltwater Flushes—These flushes have been done for thousands of years, and some health conscious individuals perform them weekly or monthly as a method of detoxification. Unless you are diagnosed with kidney disease, heart disease, or high blood pressure, saltwater flushes are generally safe, although they frequently cause nausea.

However, saltwater flushes don't work the same for everyone. Some people can't keep saltwater down. Some people's bodies absorb all the water rather than passing it through, thereby gaining extra water weight and storing extra salt.

Drinking water with a pinch of high quality sea salt offers many healthful benefits. To me, it's very different than chugging down 32 ounces of saltwater while my body protests. However, some people love saltwater flushes, and it is their go-to colon cleanse. To perform a saltwater flush, combine two teaspoons of sea salt with 32 ounces of warm water.

Drink the entire solution within 15-20 minutes. Then, sit or walk until you feel the urge to use the bathroom (10 minutes to half-hour). Be sure to follow this with sugar-free electrolytes to prevent dehydration, muscle cramps, and weakness.

2. DIY At-Home Enemas

Warm Water Enemas—Our grandmothers and great-grandmothers often used home enemas to relieve a fever and calm an upset stomach or asthma attack. Home enemas are basically self-administered colon cleanses. They can be done using water, aloe vera juice, wheatgrass, coffee, or herbal teas such as chamomile, slippery elm, chaparral, and essential oils. Enemas help flush toxins initiated by a detoxifying fast, so it's good for everyone to know how to do one.

When you fast, you want to make sure that your bowels are emptying, just as they would if eating solid food. Going a day without a bowel movement is not good, and many people don't have one if they're only drinking fluids and not eating fiber-rich foods. It's a wonderful treatment to give yourself an at-home enema when you're fasting, cleansing, or even when you're just not feeling well or your energy is low. I also know from first hand experience that in certain circumstances an at-home enema can also relieve a headache in no time, so it's worth a try (see Resource Guide).

Coffee Enemas—This can be a game changer for health and ageless beauty. Toxins in the liver, from stress as well as the environment, ravage the skin. Coffee enemas can brighten our skin and reduce wrinkles, plus be a powerful tool for reducing chronic pain and inflammation.

We owe the popular use of coffee enemas to Dr. Max Gerson, who developed a technique for liver detoxification called Gerson Therapy. In a story that Charlotte Gerson tells in her book about her father's work, the usage of coffee enemas dates back to World War I.

Severely wounded soldiers were sent back from the front lines in need of surgery, yet little anesthetic was available. Nurses often gave enemas to the soldiers immediately prior to or following surgery. The story goes that one day a nurse accidentally poured coffee into her patient's enema bag instead of water. The pain relief supposedly experienced by the soldiers was so profound that it is said this became a regular practice with the surgical nurses.

Whether rumors or reports coming from the front, two doctors at the German University of Goettingen's College of Medicine later studied the phenomena by injecting coffee into the rectum of mice and found that it caused the bile ducts to open.

Dr. Max Gerson, having learned of the studies with rats by Dr. O. A. Meyer and Professor Martin Heubner, MD, began his own experiment at home. He claimed they relieved his migraine headaches. Then, Dr. Gerson went on to develop a protocol of enemas. Gerson Therapy includes a specific diet to treat diseases such as cancer, as well as anxiety and depression. Learn more about coffee enemas in the Resource Guide. If caffeine-sensitive, substitute chlorophyll for coffee.

3. Professional Colonics

Professional colonics can be an ideal self gift. Administered in a serene spa-like setting by a licensed hydrocolonic therapist, these can be both relaxing and rejuvenating for the mind, body, and spirit. Colonics, however, are an intimate procedure, involving body parts we do not generally talk about with other people. A colon therapist's most important job is to make the client feel safe by providing a soothing, sterile space, plus confidentiality and trust. If you arrive feeling achy, fatigued, or depressed, you are likely to leave feeling like you're on *cloud nine*; lighter physically and emotionally, as if walking on air. That's the power of cleansing the colon.

Conclusion

Colon cleansing supports the body and aids Mother Nature in building what the Braggs call "Vital Force," or energy, by lifting the dangerous weight of toxicity from overburdened organs. Paul Bragg and Patricia Bragg were among early health experts to comprehend consequences of "internal toxic poisoning, or autointoxication," as they termed it in their trailblazing manifesto on detoxification, *Miracle of Fasting*. In their characteristically bold, straight talking fashion, they summed up the problem and the solution.

"Sickness and premature aging are no mystery. If food is stuffed into an overloaded digestive tract, it rots, putrefies, and poisons your body's trillions of cells. The secret of health can be summed up in three words, 'Keep clean inside!'"

Revolutionary Beauty Alyson Charles

Meet Revolutionary Beauty Alyson Charles. Rock-Star Shaman and internationally renowned speaker, she is an author, spiritual teacher, and the host of the Ceremony Circle Podcast. She has been named by the Huffington Post as a "Top Limit-Breaking Female Founder," who serves as a bridge to the wisdom of Earth-Sky (where the name Rock-Star Shaman originates).

Julia: What is beauty?

Alyson: *I feel more beautiful now than I did 20 years ago, because I feel so clear in who I am. I'm operating from a place of self honor, self-worth, and self-respect, which comes from all the work I've done on myself and walking the spiritual path, and when I'm creating healthy boundaries and healthy containers for my relationships. That is when I feel beautiful. And by no means do I get it perfect all the time! And that's OK with me, too.*

I'm gentle with myself and embrace the feminine, expansive; ancient wisdom that comes to me through my relationship with Source. I am happy with how I choose to walk this path and experience life, so I feel like, yes, I'm a beautiful creature.

The feminine allows for inspiration, unexpected, and infinite growth and magic. When I lead from my feminine side, I am consciously creating safety for myself and my team. The feminine is expansive; it's where the infinite miracles live.

My work in this life as a Rock-Star Shaman, is to be a bridge between Rock, which is Earth; and Great Spirit and Source, which is the Star. When that name came through, I did a lot of work around making sure it was not coming from ego—

many ceremonies and rituals. I know now that I'm a bridge between worlds, and also a bridge introducing shamanism to the mainstream masses a lot through media channels and to anyone who leans into it.

I'm excited that my calling actually aligns with a way of being of service, that the older I get, the more respected I may be in our culture. Ours is a very different culture than one where elders are seen as beautiful for the ancient wisdom they carry and the path they walked.

Julia: Was there a pivotal experience that changed your life?

Alyson: *I had a spiritual awakening around the dire need for a previous relationship to end. Because I kept not listening to my body, in a nutshell, I was brought to my knees. I surrendered. I said to Source, to my guides, "I need your help. Show me the way." Before awakening, my identity was as a national champion long-distance runner, and a TV talk show and radio host. I let go of all of that. I let myself stay open to all the messages I received, and lived my life by the call, open even to things that were scary or made no sense. That is how I live my life now, every moment.*

Julia: How did you care for your body?

Alyson: *My physical body has gone through so much deep work. I was celibate for five years and it was even longer before I was in a relationship. The piece I had to heal was to learn to trust myself that I could be in a physical and intimate relationship, and not let my body be used or tormented, or dishonored.*

My dad was my running coach, and I pushed my body beyond its limit on a daily basis from the time I was three when I was in my first race! But my relationship with my body was one of dysfunction and disconnection. There was no time or softness, for rest.

"What is the feminine?" I asked as I was healing. I had no idea since I had been forcing my body to perform at the highest levels for so long. The relationship to my body and my worth was about what it could perform. Softness and femininity were foreign essences.

My definition of the feminine is to live by the call, by feeling into my belly. It's learning how to trust and that you can lead with softness, love, and kindness. Trust is a big one.

Julia: What purification practices did you use as you were awakening your body and spirit?

Alyson: *Before my awakening, when my body was clamoring to get my attention, saying "You are really offtrack; you are not living your dharma at all," one of the things that came through was to drink fresh organic vegetable juices and get colonics. I love colon hydrotherapy. I am a huge believer. I attribute colonics to helping me get in touch with my emotional body. It was a huge catalyst for my awakening!*

MODULE 3

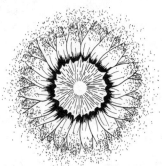

EPISODE 6
CLEAN DEEP, GLOW BRIGHT & NEVER DIET AGAIN

"The greatest discovery by modern man is the method to rejuvenate himself physically, mentally, and spiritually by fasting. We can create a quality of agelessness and ignite our body's Vital Force to heal any illness or disease."

—Paul Bragg and Patricia Bragg, *Miracle of Fasting*

Patricia Bragg credits her radiant health, beautiful skin, slim figure, and unstoppable energy to routinely fasting one day a week for all of her adult life. The *Miracle of Fasting*, written by her father Paul Bragg in 1966, and later revised by Patricia in 1972, is considered *The Fasting Bible*. This guide is the foundation of the Bragg Healthy Lifestyle.

If you attempted to fast and felt weak, hungry, light-headed, or nauseated, and unable to continue, do not be intimidated! The Revolutionary Beauty fasting protocol will arm you with the tricks and tools to safely fast without discomfort. While the *Miracle of Fasting* recommends a water fast, I have found fasting with green vegetable juice as effective for purification. This method protects blood sugar balance. For those who find fasting with water or juices impossible for health reasons, immense benefits can be achieved by utilizing nutritious drinks. Some of these are organic smoothies, bone broths, and detoxifying soups. I coined the term *Fasting Lite* to describe this gentle cleansing method. This allows nearly anyone to give their body a rest from digestion, which takes more energy than almost any physical activity!

Creating Renewable Energy and Why We Age

Aging is directly connected to the body's ability to renew trillions of cells. Nothing regenerates the body's cells like fasting. This practice improves sleep, boosts energy, and decreases the risk of illness. You will feel like a new person because rapid cell renewal is literally recreating your body.

Due to a toxic environment, cells age faster than ever. More than two billion pounds of pesticides are dumped onto America's farmlands each year. Genetically modified foods (GMOs) are indigestible. Cancer rates have skyrocketed since the introduction of GMOs into the food chain. Monsanto's use of Glycophosphate, the main ingredient in the herbicide, Roundup, coincides with an unprecedented spike in cancer, infertility, birth defects, autoimmune diseases, asthma, and viruses. The percentage of wheat allergies and sensitivities has increased by 40 percent in children and adults in the last two decades.

These toxins are assimilated into the system through food, air, beauty, and cleaning products. Without proper elimination, these toxins are stored in the body and brain forever, unless we internally cleanse. *Internal cleansing* includes dry-skin brushing, lymphatic drainage massage, and organ detoxification.

Autointoxication describes the state of being poisoned by toxic substances within the body. Patricia Bragg writes that "Autointoxication is the greatest enemy of vibrant health.

It's the root cause of all major physical troubles because illness starts in a poisoned bloodstream. Autointoxication is the basis of most troubles that affect the heart, liver, kidneys, and joints. When our bloodstream and lymphatic system— your river of life—becomes poisoned, this has more to do with premature aging than all the other causes combined."

Igniting the Inner Healer

As a professional colon therapist, gut health expert, and fasting coach, I have seen this truth in action. The *inner healer* is always present in the body, ready to build Vital Force, even when the mind is overcome with fear—another side effect, ironically, of neurotoxins in the food chain. Flushing these toxins through fasting is the most effective way to reverse aging. With this, you may feel a vibrancy you have not experienced in years.

Many find that one of the most potent experiences of fasting is mental clarity. This is why fasting has been used by sages and spiritual teachers since the beginning of time. As you become comfortable with fasting, you may use this type of cleansing as a tool when confronting a problem, experiencing loss or change, or looking for an answer to a burning question.

Intermittent Fasting

You may also want to experiment with a trending form of fasting, called *intermittent fasting*. This was introduced by Paul and Patricia Bragg in the 1970s. Intermittent fasting calls for only liquids after dinner, with no solid food until noon the next day. While many Americans were nibbling gooey donuts with sprinkles and sipping coffee with sugar and cream for breakfast, Patricia Bragg was playing a fast game of tennis. She did not dive into her first meal until lunchtime.

The reason we feel weak or experience headaches when we fast is due to autointoxication. As a result, we feel tired, achy, and cranky. Most of these detox symptoms are avoidable. When we prepare for a fast with the cleansing and detoxification protocols discussed, as well as salt baths and saunas, the result is a pain-free and enjoyable fast. Without these cleansing rituals, we are pushing poison from one part of the body to another. Master healer and naturopath, Dr. Robert Cass, refers to this as "moving deck chairs on the Titanic."

The secret to comfortable fasting is to take advantage of simple detoxification protocols. The reason people feel fabulous at detoxification spas is due to the expert cleansing methods available. Sure, they are removed from their normal, stressful environment and the enticement of special occasions. However, the cleansing support services offered eliminate and greatly reduce detoxification symptoms. We Care in Desert Hot Springs, California, even offers safe daily colonics to their fasters. You can do the same thing, right in your own home.

Fasting will likely become one of the most enjoyable experiences you will create for yourself. Expect crazy amounts of energy, crystal clear mental acuity, and even weight loss. Experience a lightness and lose the belly bloat. Patricia Bragg has never dieted. She doesn't believe in counting calories. Her weekly fast—and seasonal 4-7 day cleanses—have kept her body sleek and sensational for decades. Fasting ignites your engine, literally, by turbocharging the metabolism. When you integrate detoxification protocols such as dry skin brushing and colon cleansing, you flush accumulated toxins stored in fat cells. When these poisons are released during fasting, weight loss is inevitable. Watch the cellulite and puffiness dissipate!

Electrolytes, the Energy of Life

Electrolyte minerals are the energy of life. Minerals such as sodium, potassium, and magnesium conduct electricity throughout the body. We lose electrolytes while in stressful situations or exercising. Detoxification also flushes electrolytes—energy is boosted during fasts and cleanses upon replacement of electrolytes. We recommend sugar-free electrolyte supplementation during a fast. Electrolytes prevent dehydration. They buffer acids that certain foods and body functions create. This maintains the body's optimal pH balance. Without this balance, we do not absorb nutrients. Without nutrients, we are actually starving ourselves to death.

When the body cannot maintain proper acid-alkaline pH, the system will find a way to restore balance. Electrolyte buffers from the cells are depleted, and minerals leech from bones. We use large amounts of calcium and magnesium to neutralize this imbalance. No wonder so many struggle with osteoporosis and osteoarthritis!

Fasting alkalizes the body more quickly and proficiently than any other protocol—including the attempt to maintain a *perfect diet*. Add in stress—an unavoidable component of life—and acid levels skyrocket. Live blood cell analysis reveals that stress makes twice the impact on creating acidity in the digestive system as food. In addition to the stress busting exercises we've discussed earlier, fasting is one of the safest and easiest ways to push the emotional reset button. Think of fasting—in whatever form you choose—as a safety net. One day a week, the cells will use their energy for rest and regeneration instead of digestion.

Stress and Acidity

Stress produces acidity not only in the stomach but throughout the body. We burn more electrolytes on a stressful day, than from a five-mile run. This is why many women who eat a wholesome diet cannot balance their pH and experience the physical and emotional symptoms of over-acidity. These include low energy, belly bloat, and sagging skin. Over-acidity depletes the minerals that calm nerves as well as bolster patience and creativity. This leaves us feeling cranky and tired, with less ability to solve problems.

Both dehydration and over-acidity, which often occur to-gether, can mimic the symptoms of a blood sugar crash—brain fog, headache, and fatigue. The next time you feel the *4 pm crash*, drink a large glass of electrolyte infused water. You will feel better. If you don't, reach for a protein smooth-ie—and forgo the chips!

The Acid and Alkaline Balance

You may have heard of the body's delicate acid-alkaline bal-ance and want to know how pH affects your health. The body is alkaline by nature, but acid forms as we ingest acidic foods such as meat, eggs, and grains. As the body breathes, moves, and digests, our system creates acid. In other words, the body must always maintain alkalinity. Yet, every bodily function, by necessity, creates acids. This affects health, lon-gevity, and causes premature aging of cells and skin.

The processes that power the body need acids. We can't live without them. However, the acid-alkaline balance is fre-quently disrupted. The systems that need acidity—such as digestion—do not produce enough enzymes to digest food. Alternatively, alkaline propelled, acid sensitive structures—such as the nervous system—are flooded. *That* is why we age! That is why we are sick, bloated, and depressed. Luckily, the solution is simple. Knowledge is power.

Gastric acids, including hydrochloric acid (HCL), combine in the stomach with foods, liquids, and digestive enzymes to process foods. When this happens effectively, energizing nu-trients are released into the bloodstream and organs. Diges-tive enzymes occur naturally in a properly functioning stom-ach, as well as in saliva and the intestines. Combined with the mucus coating of the stomach and intestines, HCL helps elim-inate harmful bacteria to protect the body from infection.

A leading cause of illness and chronic pain is over-acidity. In addition to stress, this imbalance is caused by specific foods—especially processed and fast-foods.

An imbalance in acid and alkaline levels may cause:

- Brain fog
- Joint pain
- Low energy
- Weight gain
- Muscle cramps
- Dry, lifeless skin
- Tension and anxiety
- Hormone imbalance
- Infertility and menopausal discomfort

Serious results of an imbalanced pH in the body can lead to:

- Cancer
- Immune breakdown
- Stressed liver function
- Cardiovascular disease
- Pancreatic dysfunction
- Bladder and kidney disease
- Yeast overgrowth and candida

One of the best ways to create and maintain balanced acid-alkalinity is through diet. While even some organic foods—including grains, meat, and eggs, are acidic, we can balance this by consuming sparingly. Pairing acidic foods with alkaline foods also supports a harmonious acid-alkaline balance.

Alkaline foods:

- Herbs
- Beans
- Herbal teas
- Unsalted butter
- Organic bone broth
- Most fruits, including citrus
- Millet, quinoa, and amaranth
- Potassium-rich vegetable broth
- Most vegetables—especially greens
- *Super food* greens such as spirulina and wheatgrass

The following foods produce acidity:

- Soda
- Sugar
- Meats
- Cheese
- Peanuts
- Fast-foods
- Egg whites
- Fried foods
- Salted butter
- Processed foods
- Coffee and black tea
- Refined vegetable oils
- Grains, especially wheat and wheat products

One to two weeks before your first fast, choose a highly alkaline diet. Add green vegetable juices, sugar-free electrolyte drinks, and apple cider vinegar drinks to your meal plan.

Alkalizing the Body with Apple Cider Vinegar

Paul and Patricia Bragg introduced apple cider vinegar to America. Yes, they *wrote the book* on that, too.

Although acetic acid, the primary component of apple cider vinegar (ACV) is acidic, the effect on the body is alkalizing. This is the perfect antidote to balance pH levels and detoxify your bloodstream. In their best-selling book, *Apple Cider Vinegar Miracle Health System*, Paul and Patricia Bragg write: "Natural, organic, raw ACV can be called one of Mother Nature's most perfect foods, the world's first natural medicine. Natural ACV is a rich light golden color and held to the light, you might see a tiny formation of *cobweb-like* substances we call the ... 'mother.'"

This miracle "mother" is the unprocessed, unpasteurized, unfiltered apple cider from which vinegar is made. This appears cloudy, and may even contain small amounts of sediment, similar to fresh pressed organic apple juice. However, this elixir contains a culture of beneficial bacteria produced by the acidulation process. That is why ACV never needs refrigeration.

Acetic acid has been shown to lower cholesterol, reduce blood pressure levels, and improve heart health. The following are just a few of the hundreds of uses for ACV:

- Reduces seasonal allergies
- Balances blood sugar levels
- Relieves symptoms of acid reflux and heartburn
- Stimulates metabolism and increases weight loss
- Relieves pain in the joints caused by acid crystals and diseases such as arthritis
- Boosts the body's immunity with antibacterial and antifungal properties
- Supports gut health by adding a healthy dose of bacteria to the digestive system
- Purifies all organs; flushes toxins from the kidneys and liver, phlegm from the lungs and lymphatic system

To begin using ACV, add one teaspoon to eight ounces of water and drink twice daily. You may add a touch of honey, or monk fruit powder (zero glycemic) for sweetening. If you feel detoxification symptoms upon drinking—such as headache or nausea—be patient. This will pass as your organs detoxify. Slowly work up to one teaspoon of ACV mixed with just one tablespoon of water before each meal. Some people use as much as one tablespoon twice daily.

Some uses that are uniquely relevant to create ageless renewable energy:

- ACV is a wonderful skin toner and facial cleanser. Dilute a cotton ball with equal parts water and ACV— then, pat gently onto your face and body.
- ACV is healing for sunburns and scar tissue and can help dissolve a long-standing scar within months.

The Miracle of Wheatgrass

Wheatgrass juice has been an integral part of my healing journey, as well as for millions of others. I discovered this green drink as my modeling career faltered, derailed by recurrent health issues that called for radical solutions. My first husband, David, read Dr. Ann Wigmore's *The Wheatgrass Book* in 1980. Inspired, he turned our tiny studio into a wheatgrass greenhouse. My body was so filled with toxins that I could only take one teaspoon at a time without becoming violently ill. Within six months, I was able to drink eight ounces a day—a practice to which I have been dedicated ever since.

The transformation I experienced as I integrated wheatgrass and colon cleansing into my life led David and I to study with Dr. Wigmore at Hippocrates Health Institute. We witnessed the magic of wheatgrass for cell renewal and regeneration. My asthma disappeared for good, as did the migraines. Because wheatgrass is only one molecule different from human blood, no wonder this substance is so powerful. Wheatgrass is a potent anti-inflammatory, antibacterial, and antifungal. You will not find a stronger antioxidant in Mother Nature. Begin slowly, with no more than an ounce on an empty stomach. Wheatgrass does not provoke wheat sensitivities.

Dr. Wigmore and our fearless leader, Patricia Bragg, were twin souls in many ways. Both tiny in stature, but mighty, and devoted to their ministry—the message of health and healing. Like Patricia, Dr. Ann did not care that people thought of them as kooks or eccentrics. They understood that the simple principles of Mother Nature are profoundly restorative.

Action Steps

1. Measure Your pH

Keep a diary of your body's pH as you go through the Revolutionary Beauty program. It's easy to measure your pH by buying pH strips online or at any drug or health food store.

Merely pee on the stick to instantly see your acid or alkaline level measured by color. Colors are coded on the package within ranges from acidity to alkalinity. The desired range is from 6.4-7.4—which may vary throughout the day. A good habit is to take a daily measurement until pH is balanced.

2. Add sugar-free electrolytes to your diet daily

Electrolytes can be a game changer for boosting your energy, clearing brain fog, strengthening your bones, and lifting your spirit. Buy water charged with electrolytes, or purchase sugar-free powdered or liquid electrolytes to mix with bottled water. We have been led to believe that only athletes need extra electrolytes, but we all do, especially busy women! And what woman do you know who isn't busy?

3. Track your trace minerals

Take a trace mineral supplement and a magnesium supplement. This will support your electrolyte supply, aid in bowel regularity, and calm your mind, which makes it easier to release stress and tension.

Detoxification flushes electrolytes—replacement during fasts, boosts energy. We recommend sugar-free electrolyte supplementation during your fast to prevent dehydration. These buffer the acids that certain foods and bodily functions create. This maintains the body's optimal acid-alkaline balance.

Revolutionary Beauty Kelly LeBrock

Actress and supermodel, Kelly LeBrock, began her career at 16 and starred in a 24-page spread for *Vogue Magazine* at 19. One of her most recognizable roles was the gorgeous face in the Pantene shampoo ad with the tagline, "Don't Hate Me Because I'm Beautiful," which became a pop culture catchphrase. Cast as the *perfect* or *fantasy* woman in the films *Women in Red* and *Weird Science*, she was for decades considered one of Hollywood's sexiest women.

As beautiful on the inside as she is exquisite on the outside, we met when she came for a colon hydrotherapy session which followed her fast at Optimal Health Spa in San Diego, California. Kelly left her career in Hollywood in the early 1990s to move to a Santa Ynez ranch and devote herself to motherhood. Raising three children who own her heart, she is rediscovering the wild spirit that has always lived inside her.

Julia: When did you find radical self-care?

Kelly: *I went to a spa in Mexico when I was 19, and I have always looked into different medicines aside from the conventional. I'm attracted to eastern medicine, and I think that comes from my love of nature, and I've done fasts and cleanses for 35 years. One of the first, and one of the most amazing, was the Master Cleanse—lemon juice, maple syrup, and cayenne— which I did for 14 days. I went off food for three days first and went straight into just liquid. I did that in Indonesia. I had just had a baby, and I decided to do a cleanse. I was so clear that I felt as if I was talking to God. I went beyond hunger and I was connecting to feelings and thoughts I didn't know were there. I never wanted to eat again!*

As for wheatgrass, I have had a love-hate relationship with wheatgrass for 35 years, but, Julia, your passion for it is contagious! So I'm doing it again. I learned about it a long time ago, and read how doctors would recommend it. Back in the day, when I first started, I overdid it at first and had all kinds of reactions—cleansing reactions such as headaches and body aches from all the toxins pouring into my bloodstream. Of course, being me, I drank way too much of it. So people have to be careful, start slow. It does move things around in your body and in your bowels. I want to say one thing: I know you like to put celery in it, but when it's cold and damp, you don't want cold things, you want warm things, so add ginger, OK? As for beauty, to me, beauty is wildness. It is warmth and radiance; it is embracing the light and the dark. Because I was considered attractive, no one cared to know what was inside of me, who I really was. So, I focused on that, on becoming a person I like and respect, and it took decades! When I moved into the wilderness, I discovered real beauty, and that is who I am in nature, as a part of everything wild and alive.

Wild is a very important thing, a very intimate thing, I think. I am the archetypal woman, not male or female; I am in between. I don't distinguish between gender. I fall in love with souls; I got sick and tired of being spit on, and when those things keep happening, you have to look at yourself and say, "What is going on?" Maybe that's a revolution of sorts.

Julia: Motherhood, what has that been for you?

Kelly: It's been the most incredible, crazy, wonderful, magical journey. I quit my career; some women do both; I didn't want both. I wanted to be present for them. Today they are all incredible, selfless, kind, generous heart thinking people. I am truly grateful. They say I'm lucky; I worked hard, I worked fucking hard! It's not easy cleaning up tears that have been spilled because of situations that you can't control. They have a real work ethic and live very real lives.

Julia: Did you experience abuse in your past?

Kelly: Early on, yes, very early on. The first few times that were really violent, I was about 15 or so. I suffered silently, and then, I was propelled into this fake world of smoke and mirrors. I have often wondered what the world be like if we didn't have mirrors.

I believe that when we look in the mirror, what we see in the mirror is not what other people see. I think there are two ways of seeing, and you have to be conscious of the way you perceive yourself. I do have mirrors, and I try to look at myself in them in pure light, and not be critical.

What is real is how we see ourselves when we look in the pond. Our reflection in a pond is true beauty, because there is movement and ripples and changes; it's soft and safe. When we look *in a mirror, it's mercury's idea of what we look like—it can be cold and stark.*

Maybe when some people see me, they see glamour. But I am a pure peasant at heart, a girl with dirt under my nails. If you can't have dirt under your nails, you will never have true love in your heart. You learn self-respect or you die. There is an emotional death that happens when you're in a revolution of self. I think that comes from having time and peace to look inside, and not be afraid anymore.

I looked up what revolution means: the true meaning is "a very sharp change," and I think a sharp change had to happen or I would not be around. If you don't find those great magnetic positive polarities to pull yourself out of the abyss, then you can't help yourself, and you can't help those around you.

What saved me was helping others. When you have been such a big face, a big voice, a big body, and yet no one has heard your screams, a change has to happen. I believe there is a deafening cry within women who have been abused or battled trauma, where we have we go inside and listen to our own heart. If we come out on the other end, we are amazing people.

Real beauty regimes comes from inside; you can buy the creams but they won't do anything if you don't care for your whole body. Beauty comes from what you eat, what you feel, what you speak, and what you see.

If you bring the demons to the table and look them in the eye, they cannot hurt you. I have run from them, but I discovered healing comes when you sit with them. I have fought for every breath I take, and I fight for others, too.

We are all in this together.

MODULE 3

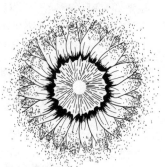

Episode 7
THE SKINNY ON
SUCCESSFUL FASTING

"Fasting is the greatest remedy, the physician within."

—Paracelsus, 15th century Physician,
Alchemist, and Body Chemistry Pioneer

Pre-Fasting Protocol

Let's make your first fast a win! This simple protocol flushes toxins even before you trade your pasta for a shot of wheatgrass juice. Before you begin a fast, we recommend that you prepare. Reduce the following items for one to two weeks:

- Dairy
- Sugar
- Alcohol
- Wheat
- Red meat

- Sodas
- Fake fats
- Junk food
- Fried food
- Processed food

Wean yourself from them slowly. If you are a coffee drinker, reduce intake as much as possible. Enjoy slightly caffeinated green tea or matcha, which rebalances rather than energizes. America's most popular coffee substitute, the highly alkaline Teeccino, was created by Revolutionary Beauty Caroline MacDougall. Enjoy this delicious treat!

Coffee and black tea are acidic. Over-acidity, as we know, dries and wrinkles our skin and stiffens our joints. To diminish the discomfort of coffee withdrawals, do a water enema, (or better yet, a coffee enema) or colonic. You will instantly feel better. We like to say the best use of coffee is in a colonic!

Movement and Fasting

Light exercise is recommended as part of your fasting protocol. Exercise moderately during a fast; try a light jog rather than a five-mile run, or gentle yoga instead of hot yoga. Pilates and resistance stretching are excellent. Bouncing on the rebounder moves the lymph. Pay attention to your body's signals. Hydrate, hydrate, hydrate!

During your fast, you may feel exhilarating amounts of energy. While this is morale boosting, don't overdo it by staying up late or cleaning the whole house! Let your body use this energy for purification. This attention to detoxification shifts the deeper programming that insists we must always be busy. Detoxification and healing are worthy uses of your energy. If you feel inclined to create, do something special just for you. Catch your dreams in a journal. Listen to the voice that may be buried in to-do lists. She deserves to be heard. Fasting unlocks the unconscious where our true self lives.

Your Fasting Day

For your first fast, clear your calendar. Once fasting becomes a regular ritual, you will be able to do anything that you normally do. You may experience symptoms of withdrawal—such as headaches, body aches, nausea, or brain fog. This is why relying on the protocols listed will save you discomfort.

Detoxification Protocols

The following detoxification protocols support your body as your system purges toxins throughout your fast. They will also reduce hunger and eliminate cravings. You will feel lighter and brighter.

The protocols below will reduce detoxification symptoms:

- Salt baths and saunas
- Hot shower followed by cold shower
- Dry skin brushing and lymphatic drainage therapy
- Colon cleansing—including herbal teas, flaxseed flushes, enemas, and colonics

If an underlying health condition needs attention, contact a professional. In collaboration with your doctor, you might also consider a series of professional colon hydrotherapy treatments to forge a deeper level of detoxification. After all, toxicity and stress are the two main sources of illness and disease. Today's functional medicine doctors are well versed in the importance of purification for physical and mental health (see Resource Guide).

The Ritual of Fasting

"The CARE Plan" suggests one 24-hour fast every week, or a constant routine of intermittent fasting—16 consecutive hours while eating only during eight hours of the day. The more you fast, the easier fasting becomes. You may discover while fasting that your body needs much less food than you are accustomed to eating. All long-lived people—such as the famous Hunzas of the Himalayas—consume less food than most Americans. Fasting retrains the brain to be satisfied with less, and lust for fresh fruits and vegetables rather than hamburgers and french fries. Fasting has maintained Patricia's weight—which is the same now as when she was 40. While traveling the globe, if she could not find fresh food,

Patricia would fast rather than eat junk. If this seems an impossible goal, over time and with weekly fasts, you may surprise yourself. Through the practice of fasting, the concept of calories and pounds becomes obsolete.

Fasting Lite and Liquid Nutrition

For those who would like to experience the physical and mental liberation of fasting, but cannot fast on juice or water, you can detoxify safely by *Fasting Lite*. That describes consuming liquid nourishment such as smoothies and clear or blended soups for a day or more. Fasting Lite is wonderful for lifting energy and spirit while nourishing the body with protein, and a balanced amount of carbohydrates, if you wish. Add ample vegetable juice to boost nutrient levels.

Although not a classic fast, the benefits Fasting Lite yields are immense. Cleansing and purification take many forms. One plan does not work well for all person. Fasting Lite accommodates a variety of health and lifestyle issues and is an introduction to fasting itself.

Fasting Grocery List

- Two quarts organic vegetable juices
- An abundance of fresh, pure water
- Blended vegetable soups and organic bone broth
- Sugar-free, gluten-free, dairy-free protein powders, mixed with water or non-dairy milk
- Smoothies made with low-sugar fruits (fresh or frozen, such as berries) and veggies (fresh or frozen, such as spinach and kale)
- Optional: Wheatgrass juice
- Optional: Herbal teas, fresh, or frozen chlorophyll

Be sure to incorporate as many of the same detoxification protocols as a regular fast calls for:

- Colon cleansing
- Dry skin brushing
- Lymphatic drainage therapy
- Hot and cold showers saunas

Although you will be taking in nutrients, you may still experience detoxification symptoms such as headaches or fatigue from eliminating coffee, sugar, processed foods, alcohol, and anything you find yourself craving—even bread or pasta. Sugar and carbohydrates are the source of most cravings!

Fasting Lite is a fabulous way to reduce the use of toxic substances, wielding the energy and mental focus to do the tasks you need to do.

Longer Fasting

Once you have become comfortable with routine fasting, you may choose a longer fast. Fasting Lite can be done safely for five, seven, and even up to 30 days. However, we suggest that you reach out to a fasting coach or health professional for any fast longer than five days. Just as you see emblazoned across your television screen "Do Not Try This at Home. These are Professionals!" while watching a stunt driver fly a truck over ten flaming cars—the same is true for long fasts. *We don't know what we don't know!*

Fasting is an ancient, deep, and potent healing process, humbling on every level. Universally, indigenous people participated in fasts and cleanses led by a shaman, a medicine woman or man. They helped prepare and condition fasters. Give yourself and your body the same due respect.

Longer fasts assist in the release of addictions and cravings, as well as help heal:

- Anxiety
- Depression
- Food allergies
- Environmental allergies

Fasting for 10-14 days each January has dramatically reduced my spring hay fever. If you are healthy and have done 24-hour fasts, you can safely fast on your own for 2-5 days.

Breaking Your Fast

Your first post-fast meal should be light and clean, such as fresh fruit, a small salad, or a healthy smoothie. That first bite will taste uniquely delicious! You may feel full sooner than usual. Acknowledge your body's experience of satiety and use this opportunity to transition to smaller meals of whole foods. This takes time and practice. Decade-long habits do not disappear overnight, and conditioning runs deep. Memories of sweet, salty, and fatty foods equal feelings of love and warmth for many people.

I've heard dozens of tales from clients who broke their fast with Thanksgiving dinner, or birthday cake and champagne. This unfortunate choice was often followed by a night on the porcelain throne. When we cleanse, we become more sensitive to toxic foods. The origin of the word "celebrate" is the Latin word *celebrare*, to honor. Can we learn to honor our bodies, souls, and spirits with pure, clean food? Absolutely, with time, practice, and patience.

Intermittent Fasting

Paul Bragg introduced intermittent fasting, which he called the "No Breakfast Plan." Now a popular lifestyle choice, intermittent fasting means consuming no solid food past 7 pm (after dinner) until noon or lunch the next day. Patricia Bragg has been an intermittent faster all her life. I have enjoyed this practice for the last 22 years, which always fills me with energy and a buoyant spirit.

Intermittent fasting is based on the understanding that our bodies need at least 12 hours to digest, cleanse, and repair. If this ritual sounds too daunting, you might add a protein smoothie, bone broth, or herbal tea to your morning ritual. You may do the same if you stay awake late.

While intermittent fasting is beloved by many, this practice may not work for you. No one way of eating or living works for everyone. Consequently, what works during one season of life may not work in another. Intermittent fasting suits those who never crave a large meal at breakfast.

What about coffee? Though many well-known intermittent fasting coaches support coffee as the morning *drink of choice*, the acidity adds years to the skin. If healthy, with no history of breast congestion or cysts, enjoy coffee as a once a day treat, if you like. Yet, a better choice for a morning beverage is green tea, white tea, or matcha.

Use Fasting to Discover Your Perfect Diet

One of the best reasons to fast is to experience ultimate health and happiness—how living in our bodies could feel. On the flip side, fasting may show what foods do not agree with you. Right after a fast, uncomfortable feelings such as gas or bloating are easier to notice than at any other time.

The optimal way to reintroduce foods after a fast is to add them one at a time, a few days apart. We suggest you keep a food diary, to track patterns or symptoms, such as low energy and brain fog. Fasting also boosts the ability to maintain a clean diet, by reinforcing a sense of lightness and joy.

The body and mind arc to healing—with the capacity to renew and regenerate. All we need is a little support and the desire to heal.

Food Cravings and Addictions

If you struggle with food addictions or cravings, fasting is one of the most effective tools for curbing your attraction to unhealthy substances, permanently. Fasting flushes toxic substances, such as sugar and fried foods from your system, eliminating their grip on body and mind.

If you have struggled with any type of dependency—sugar, coffee, alcohol, or drugs—you know what I mean. You could swear that the devil lives in your body and has total control. That explains one of the reasons that rehabilitation centers fail for four out of five people. Lack of willpower is not the issue. Our bodies desire what is familiar.

When we cleanse, we let go of the residue of these substances so they no longer are a familiar part of us. Their release becomes effortless—we are not *white knuckling it*. We no longer wrestle with the attraction to that substance. The body, mind, and spirit are free. Like letting go of a toxic relationship, when we finally muster the courage to walk out the door, we reclaim confidence and joy. Fasting gives us the same ability to do that with food and substances—as well as everything else not working in our lives. You will be astonished by the emotional and spiritual revelations that you experience while fasting.

The ancient gurus and sages knew what they were doing. Their example is part of why fasting is a cornerstone of the Bragg Healthy Lifestyle.

No Fail Fasting

When you begin fasting, don't punish yourself if, with the best of intentions, you bail the first afternoon. Each experience is informative—our *failures* even more so. If you adhere to detoxification protocols, fasting is much easier. One of the most powerful gifts you will ever give yourself, expect transformation on every level. One thing I have learned to trust in my forty years of practice is my client's timing, and I extend that to you. Your timing will be perfect and dictated by Source and the ancestors who travel this road with you, unseen but not unheard. They will find you in your dreams and cheer you on. You are loved.

When I first opened my clinic, I found myself frustrated with a client I will call Sol. Sol was unable to follow through on just about everything—diet, exercise, and meditation. I did not know that Sol had no close friends living in town and suffered from a deeply buried trauma. Not until years later, when he reappeared with news of a steady job and a lovely partner, did he share his past with me. He was finally able to successfully embrace the purification practices his body and soul desperately needed. The safety net he created allowed him to excel now, when he could not earlier.

For others, consistently practicing the purification processes faithfully, step-by-step, built their *spiritual bank account* and sense of self-worth—which led to success in the rest of their lives. Since you're reading this book, you are ready for change. You want to experience the life you were meant to live, and you don't want to wait one more day. You are a Revolutionary Beauty.

Action Steps

1. Write in your journal on your fasting days. Fasts may boost our metabolism, but they also turn us inward.

They are a time of spiritual insights and heightened intuition. When you wake on your fasting day, ask, "What do I want to let go of today?" Write down your dreams when you wake; use fasting days to connect with your creative, artistic side.

2. Keep a post-fast-food diary. Look for a correlation between certain foods and discomfort, pain, puffiness, or weight gain. Food sensitivities trigger all three.

3. Be gentle with your approach to fasting. It is not intended as a method of deprivation or starvation. You are "the captain of your own ship," as Patricia Bragg would say, and nobody knows your body, or your needs, as well as you do. Adapt the protocols in this book that serve you in becoming whole, happy, and healthy. Choice and discernment are what make Revolutionary Beauties who they are!

Your mind and body are capable of healing. Fasting builds Vital Force through the ignition of your inner healer. This produces infinite renewable energy, removes years from your skin, and reduces toxin related issues such as cellulite and that *tire around the middle* or *muffin top*. Your whole body will change as you fast and detoxify.

Revolutionary Beauty Caroline MacDougall

Revolutionary Beauty Caroline MacDougall, the Herbal Tea Queen, has 30 years of experience in the herbal products industry. The designer of award-winning herbal beverages for companies including The Republic of Tea, Yogi Tea, and Organic Indai, Caroline is the founder of Teeccino, America's top selling coffee alternative. She began her career developing worldwide suppliers and importing herbs for Celestial Seasonings. The idea of Teeccino came to her in a dream in the mid-1990s when she was deeply involved in rainforest preservation work in Central America. Caroline is a longtime natural lifestyle connoisseur and fasting enthusiast.

Caroline: *Purification and fasting have been part of my life for decades. I relish rituals. The practice of releasing toxins that my body, mind, and spirit wish to be liberated from is part of a seasoning ritual to which I'm devoted. Letting go, on every level, makes room for what is to come. I have a deep love for Mother Nature, and the practices that our great-great-grand- mothers passed on—fasting being one of them.*

I am endlessly curious! I think curiosity is the elixir of life. When I fast, I listen to the voice inside me that's full of questions and answers. Purification practices are intrinsic to deepening my spiritual journey. They also ground me, because my family, my friends, my home, and my work—which is my passion—are all lovely distractions that I am blessed to enjoy. But fasting is for me the journey that takes me home to myself.

MODULE 4

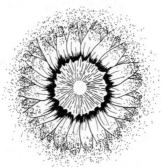

Episode 8
DIGESTION &
FOOD COMBINING

*"When diet is wrong, medicine is of no use.
When diet is correct, medicine is of no need."*

—Ayurvedic Proverb

The CARE Fueling Plan

Thousands—maybe millions—of books have been written about diet. Paul and Patricia Bragg wrote over three dozen, and I have written two. And while our fearless leader has been a vegetarian all her life, I've experimented with a variety of nutritional styles. An optimal diet is one that delights you and fills you with unstoppable energy. The perfect diet maintains ideal body weight and allows you to live craving-free—and reverses aging. Yes, with knives and forks you can turn the clock back!

The Queen of Natural Living's phrase, "No one knows what works for your body better than you," is the *golden rule for diet*. Everyone is different. No one diet works for all. Some people feel fabulous as vegans. Others require animal protein to feel their best. Paul Bragg wrote in his classic book, *Healthful Eating Without Confusion*, that ultimately the quality of food, above all other factors, is what matters. He traveled the world, observing the diets of different cultures. Some were vegetarian and others ate meat. What the healthiest people had in common was that they consumed fresh, organic food.

Given that, how does one choose their optimal diet? Let's look at the four basic principles that influence vitality and longevity:

1. Digestion—If we're not fully digesting any specific food, it is toxic to the body. We're not benefitting from the nutrients. Undigested food is recognized by the body as an allergen and causes inflammation. This in turn sends emergency responder white blood cells to fight the intruders. High levels of white blood cells have been found to be associated with high levels of body fat. When food does not digest, food turns into fat. So, the joke about a pizza going directly to our thighs is not just a joke—it's true!

2. Insulin levels—Over 85 percent of Americans are insulin resistant. That means the body is not maintaining healthy glucose levels. Insulin resistance is a main factor in heart disease and America's (and women's) number one health enemy. As functional medicine doctor and longevity expert Mark Hyman, MD, says, "This should be front-page news!" The main reason for this issue is the consumption of massive amounts of sugar. Sugar robs us of a long and pain-free life. Sugar creates the inflammation that leads to disease—diabetes is only one of them. Sugar also causes *glycation*, a fancy word for the aging of the skin!

3. Protein levels and absorption—Protein is key to insulin stability, steady energy, brain function, and

hormones. The secret to resilience, mood, and sense of optimism and joy, is protein. Most people are protein deficient. The daily protein requirement is 50-100 grams. Due to low stomach acid and other digestive issues, we may be not assimilating the protein.

Protein deficiency leads to:

- Edema
- Fatty liver
- Loss of muscle mass
- Dry skin, hair, and nails
- Out of control cravings
- Inability to lose belly fat
- Greater risk of bone fractures

4. The level of toxins—Processed food is like a freeway of dangerous chemicals, antibiotics, and hormones. The preservatives added are to ensure the longevity of the product, not humans! We choose the type of fuel that powers our vehicle. Would you fill your gas tank with liquid sugar rather than premium fuel?

However, while we understand that a green salad is healthier than a gooey donut, why do we continue to choose sugar as our body's fuel? The answer is not lack of impulse control. When the body is fed sufficient digestible protein, and other factors are addressed—especially stress—*white knuckling it* becomes a thing of the past. Revolutionary Beauties are not owned by their cravings. You will learn what this freedom feels like. If that sounds impossible, suspend your disbelief for a moment, and trust the process.

This episode will present the template for age reversal—plus share effortless maintenance tools. The respect gained when you make food your friend and overcome cravings is foundational to your self-worth. If we were granted a dollar for each hour we lectured ourselves on food choices, we would be wealthy! Food is only one facet of life, but a big one. "The CARE Fueling Plan" is simple and timeless. Science has unequivocally proven what Paul Bragg wrote about 100 years ago. Fresh, whole, organic foods regenerate minds and bodies. "The CARE Plan" embraces all lifestyle choices— vegetarian, vegan, keto, paleo, or macrobiotic.

With "The CARE Fueling Plan," your body will find its natural weight, which you will maintain effortlessly. Willpower is unnecessary. Designed to make eating joyful and nourishing, "The CARE Fueling Plan" is based on the Bragg Healthy Lifestyle with tools to eliminate cravings and improve digestion.

"The CARE Plan" offers proven suggestions to boost metabolism. Why do we continue to choose sugar as our body's fuel? You deserve a beautiful body—tummy, thighs, and bum—not one forever puffy and bloated. If you struggle to lose weight, the source may well be poor digestion.

Do you suffer from any digestive related conditions?

- IBS
- gas
- bloating
- weight gain
- diarrhea
- allergies
- brain fog
- constipation

Healthy digestion is key to energy and ageless beauty. The first step is to visit the world of digestive enzymes. Digestive enzymes are the magic bullet which protects the gut and turns food into fuel—not fat.

Digestive Enzymes: Digestion Protection

Americans visit internists for gastrointestinal issues four times more than for any other physical complaint. Digestion is everything. Vitality, mood, and longevity are determined by digestion. No number of sit-ups can flatten a gassy and bloated belly. Indeed, digestive health can.

Enzymes make digestion work. They are the biocatalysts that activate vitamins, minerals, proteins, and every other compound in the body; and essential to life.

One way to increase food enzyme levels in your stomach is to take one teaspoon of raw, organic Apple Cider Vinegar diluted in one tablespoon of water thirty minutes before meals. Another way is to take a food enzyme such as Enzyme Energy, which I created to help sensitive people digest food.

One of the secrets of digestive health and energy is food enzymes. I don't think I ever digested anything before I discovered them. I always felt bloated, gassy, and foggy headed after a meal, even a light one. Taking digestive enzymes with each meal eliminates bloat and brain fog. Each type of food requires a different food enzyme. Protein, for instance, requires HCL, or hydrochloric acid. When you eat a high protein meal, make sure your food enzyme includes low dose HCL. Many HCL supplements include up to 600 mg of HCL—a high dose which can cause stomach upset and acid reflux. This is one reason I created Enzyme Energy, a low dose, well tolerated HCL supplement.

Digestive enzymes mimic the enzymes naturally created in the gut. Food enzymes help the body assimilate the nutrients we need, and eliminate those we do not. Since gut health is the determining factor in immune system strength, food enzymes boost resistance to illness. A lack of digestive enzymes halts metabolism and sets the stage for numerous degenerative health conditions.

Do you get sleepy after you eat? A lack of digestive enzymes also affects the pancreas—the blood sugar regulator. By taking digestive enzymes, after we eat, we feel energized and clearheaded—not *blah* and bloated. The main reason this happens is that cooking destroys enzymes. The body uses a phenomenal amount of energy to digest cooked food.

Dr. Edward Howell, enzymatic research pioneer and peer of Paul Bragg, wrote in his classic book, *Enzyme Nutrition*, that man evolved on mostly raw food, even raw meat. This diet contributed over half the enzymes required for digestion. The gut was designed to supply only a piece of the enzyme puzzle. Since stress stops the gut from making enzymes, many people are enzyme deprived.

This is not meant to conclude that we must eat a raw diet, including raw meat, like our ancestors. For some, raw food is difficult to digest. When I was on a raw food diet, most of my food was juiced. Juice is easy to digest and floods the body with enzymes. The Bragg Healthy Lifestyle recommends 60-70 percent raw foods for optimal health and vitality. For those with sensitive tummies, this much fiber can be tough to process. Fresh vegetable juices deliver enzymes and nutrients without digestive stress.

The Food Combining Solution

Understanding food enzymes, plus the discovery of food combining, eased my digestive issues. At 22, I learned the theory of food combining through Judy Mazel's best seller, *The Beverly Hills Diet*. Food combining is based on the premise that the body only digests certain food groups at the same time. This is a critical component of weight loss, healing allergies, and stabilizing blood sugar. Digestive vitality also reduces inflammation and cellulite.

Mazel and Bragg followers Harvey and Marilyn Diamond (*Fit For Life*) presented food combining as a magic formula for weight loss. Desperately looking for anything to heal my relentless gas, bloating, and chronic lower backache, I found the solution—food combining! This protocol transformed my health, and this simple tool may do the same for you.

Food Combining

Based on chemistry, food combining was developed in the 1930s by Dr. Howard Hay. This principle is grounded in human evolution. We became farmers only 10,000 years ago. Before that, we were hunters and gatherers. In the morning, we may have eaten berries or wild nuts. By dinnertime, we may have collected wild greens or seeds—unless our ancestral grandfathers had some luck catching a fish, bird, or found a nest of eggs. The primal dinner table did not offer multiple courses that many of us enjoy now. Only one or two items were available. The human habit was to eat nuts with seeds and to eat meat alone. Frequently, no food was available—hence regular fasting. Complex carbohydrates, such as wheat, rice, and beans, came much later. This is why digestion is so challenged today.

To consume meat, beans, rice, salad, and fruit simultaneously seems normal. Yet, biogenetically, optimal digestion came from limited food combinations, eaten seasonally. Through the advent of farming, ranching, and food storage, combinations of foods have only become available in the last blip of human evolution.

One group of humans still express these *gut instincts*—kids. Watch a child eat, and you may well see them remove a hotdog from the bun, and eat it separately. They request pasta plain with butter—no sauce. Instead of being called *biogenetically brilliant*, we label them *picky eaters*. Although my kids loved a variety of foods, they wanted everything plain. God forbid I put a banana on the cereal! The children's gut knew better.

The crux of food combining is the awareness that different digestive enzymes process carbohydrates, proteins, fats, and fruit. For carbohydrates, we need amylase, made in the saliva for predigestion. To properly digest protein, we need HCL, produced in the stomach. If we eat these two foods, carbohydrates and proteins together—as in the classic American hamburger—we create a digestive disaster.

When these two food groups land in the stomach together, the stomach acids process the proteins while the carbohydrates ferment. This is when heartburn, belching, and gas begin. In the small intestine, the enzymes for carbohydrates work overtime because the predigested amylase is short-circuited by stomach acids.

Together with food enzymes, properly combined meals create the rocket fuel of energy and ageless beauty.

Food Combining Made Simple

Ease into food combining with these simple rules:

- Eat proteins with vegetables.
- Eat carbohydrates with vegetables and fats.
- Eat fruit alone, thirty minutes before or two hours after a meal.

Blood sugar crashes occur when food is not broken down and assimilated. Since eating many different foods at once stresses the digestive system, no wonder we're exhausted rather than exhilarated after eating. This is especially frustrating when eating healthy foods, the intention of which is energy and mental clarity. We may find that even fresh foods make us feel tired. That late afternoon coffee break becomes a critical energy booster and brain defogger. Many in our culture cannot imagine life without coffee or strong tea! This is the result of the fatigue caused by improperly combined foods.

The *icing on the cake* is weight gain. When undigested food passes through the bowel into the blood and lymphatic system, it is not recognized as food. The fermenting mixture becomes a toxic substance that the body does not recognize and cannot use—or eliminate. *Hello, poochy tummy and tire around the middle!*

The best thing to boost metabolism, which activates weight loss and energy, is to properly combine foods.

The Link Between Digestible Protein and Cravings

By now, we know that weight gain is caused by slow metabolism. That sluggish metabolism is caused, in part, by a fundamental lack of digestive enzymes. That is why taking food enzymes with each meal to ensure efficient digestion is important. Equally important is to aid digestion by eating foods in natural combinations similar to our ancestors—grains with greens, meats with nuts and seeds, and fruit as a meal.

Without sufficient digestible protein, even meditation, exercise, and biofeedback may not quiet food cravings. We need from 50-100 grams of protein per day. If an O blood type, you may need more. Consuming sufficient protein, properly combined, will satisfy hunger and quell sugar and snack cravings. Blood sugar regulation—as well as weight and hormone balance—depend on sufficient amounts of digestible protein. Peaceful sleep and crystal clear thinking are the rewards of this health practice.

Listed are the number of protein grams in these healthy foods:

- One egg, 6 grams
- Quinoa, per cup, 8 grams
- Lentils, per cup, 18 grams
- Broccoli, per cup, 6 grams
- Oatmeal, per cup, 6 grams
- Edamame, per cup, 8 grams
- Almonds, per ounce, 6 grams
- Hemp seeds, per cup, 13 grams
- Pinto beans, one cup, 17 grams

- Spinach, per cup, 5 grams
- Protein shake, 15-30 grams
- Chicken, 3 ounces, 30 grams
- Sea bass, 4 ounces, 26 grams
- Wild salmon, 4 ounces, 30 grams
- Sunflower seeds, one cup, 38 grams
- Pumpkin seeds, per 1/2 cup, 14 grams
- Dark green vegetable juice, per cup, 5-10 grams

A Note about Nuts:

While nuts are considered an excellent source of protein, they include enzyme inhibitors. Nuts and seeds stay intact until they hit the ground, and do what nature intended them to do—become trees. They were designed to pass through the bowels of animals, get pooped out, and grow! If you have trouble digesting nuts, like many do, soak them for twelve to twenty-four hours. Then, allow them to dry another twelve to twenty-four hours, so they become *sprouted nuts*. These include less fat, and are easier to assimilate since the digestive process has begun.

Vegan or Paleo? Raw or Cooked?

Whether vegan or paleo, digestible protein is critical for the blood sugar and hormone balance that creates health and happiness. Although I healed on a raw food diet—consisting mainly of juices—years in practice led me to widen my horizons. During this time, I observed that raw foods are not the only path to healing. The key to health is eating fresh, whole and organic foods, which can include meat and fish.

Everyone's body is different. Some people thrive as vegans, while others feel best consuming animal protein. No one size diet fits all. Bodies change as we age, as do needs and desires. What works at one life stage does not necessarily work in another. Learning to know the body's needs takes time. Trust your gut—literally. No one knows your body as well as you.

Disease is influenced by genetics, but is also influenced by improper digestion and elimination. A congested lymphatic system and impacted colon contribute to the body's decline. Healthy elimination is as important as the food we consume. Detoxification is key to conquering disease, and healthy skin.

Dr. Mark Hyman shared the following in his wonderful docu-series, *The Longevity Roadmap*:

"Here's what the science tells us about genetic risk: your genes load the gun, but the environment pulls the trigger. Your genes determine your predisposition, but not your destiny."

"Ninety percent of chronic disease and unhealthy aging is caused by something called our 'expose-ome,' not our ge-nome. The 'expose-ome' is the sum total of all our life inputs into our biology: our diet, first and foremost; activity, stress, sleep, relationships/connections, meaning/purpose, toxins, microbes—outside and in the gut—and allergens."

The good news is we have control over almost all of it!

Disease is also caused by toxicity, whether physical or emo-tional, which stresses the system. Mental stress is equally as dangerous to our well-being as is eating fast-food or breath-ing toxic air. The ability to release stress defines well-being, and influences the all-important sleep cycle. Inner peace se-cures happiness, creating that youthful glow. Beauty is de-termined by how we see ourselves, and how we feel.

"The CARE Fueling Plan" was created for busy people with-out endless time to spend preparing meals. You may be over-whelmed by complicated recipes, or intimidated when in the kitchen. Maybe takeout or dining at your favorite restaurant is a welcome reward after an exhausting day. The problem with eating out as a lifestyle is the high level of sodium, fake fat, and sugar. Generally, restaurants serve low quality fruits, vegetables, and protein. Very few serve organic cuisine. Although, more restaurants will serve organic food in time.

With this plan, even the most *kitchen phobic* can create a scrumptious, healthy meal, *fridge to fork* in 15-30 minutes. Our plan is safe for children and teens. Packed with energy-boosting brain food and boredom-free flexibility, these recipes embrace all healthy, fresh food lifestyles. The Revolutionary Beauty Recipe Plans respect the planet—and are irresistibly delicious!

Below is a list of "The CARE Fueling Plan" *yes foods*:

- Nut milks
- Organic fruits
- Sea vegetables
- Nutritional yeast
- Organic vegetables
- Hormone-free eggs
- Raw, organic fats and oils
- Organic raw vegetable juices
- Raw goat cheese or goat milk
- Green tea, matcha, herbal tea
- Naturally fermented vegetables
- Sugar-free, dairy-free chocolate or cocoa
- Agave, rice syrup, or monk fruit sweetener
- Purified, filtered, alkaline, or distilled water
- Beans, nuts, seeds, and whole grains (no wheat)
- Soy-free, sugar-free protein powders; rice, pea, hemp
- Organic protein; animal protein such as beef, buffalo, turkey, chicken, and wild caught fish (hormone-free, wild caught) or low soy vegan

Below are the *no foods*:

- Soda
- Sugar
- Sparkling water

- Processed foods
- Hydrogenated oils
- Commercial vinegar
- Artificial sweeteners
- Wheat and white flour
- Margarine and fake fats
- Junk foods and fast-foods
- Commercial chewing gum
- Pasteurized cow milk and cheese
- Dried fruits containing sulfur dioxide
- Luncheon meats, preserved and smoked meats

The following are the *occasional foods*, (unless you have been diagnosed with cancer, autoimmune or inflammatory disease, or breast congestion.)

- Honey
- Coffee
- Maple syrup
- Glass of organic wine
- Non GMO soy products
- Clean liquor such as tequila or vodka

Will Cravings Plague Me Forever?

Once you are sugar and junk food-free for 30 days, the physical cravings will subside. Longing for sugary, high fat foods—especially those that elicit childhood memories—is human. We can sabotage ourselves with food in subtle ways. One of my clients, an event planner, dined only on sugar-free organic foods, freshly prepared, at home. Yet, when at a party—a regular requirement of her career—she often took a bite of an hordeurve or canapé. *Voila!* Forty pounds later, she appeared in my office, frustrated and confused. How could this happen? Firstly, she was allergic to wheat. When we gobble foods to which we're allergic, inflammation and weight gain occur almost immediately—as in five pounds overnight.

Certain challenging food cravings and addictions, especially sugar and carbs, are connected to candida overgrowth. Sometimes good intention is not enough. Herbal protocols that balance gut flora and control candida are crucial additions to a healthy diet. Yet, diet alone does not heal candida. If your cravings feel uncontrollable, consult a functional medicine doctor. They can diagnose candida, food allergies, vitamin or mineral deficiencies, or hormonal imbalance. All of these cause cravings to loom out of control. Do not feel frustrated cravings do not subside overnight. Be patient and trust the reward will be worthwhile!

In Conclusion

Some basics I learned early have proven forever true:

- Sugar is toxic
- Wheat, especially American wheat, causes inflammation, making it indigestible and eliciting weight gain
- Fresh, organic food is life
- Gut health comes first—detoxification is vital to ageless health and beauty
- Digestible protein is key to regeneration and building a Vital Nerve Force

To boost metabolism and speed weight loss, focus on increased protein and veggies, rather than low-fat foods.

1. Practice daily intermittent fasting, or as Paul Bragg put it, the "No Breakfast Plan" or take only liquid nutrition for 24 hours every week.
2. Use our detoxification protocols on your fasting day to promote the release of toxins and alleviate *withdrawal* symptoms. Releasing toxins shrinks fat cells.
3. Effective digestion is key. Take raw, organic ACV first in the morning and before meals. Or, take digestive enzymes with each meal—with HCL and protein meals.

4. Practice food combining to boost metabolism, decrease gas and bloating, increase energy, and allow your body to find its perfect weight.

5. Consume 50-100 grams of digestible protein each day; use protein shakes in between meals or when on-the-go to stave off sugar cravings.

6. Vegetable juices and protein smoothies are optimal nutrient dense, natural fast-foods.

7. Never leave home without packing a protein shake or healthy snack.

8. Choose organic whenever possible.

Exercises

For this episode, your *exercises* are to practice at home our "CARE Fueling Plan" outlined in this episode. And, to make it easy, we are thrilled to share the luscious, simple recipes of licensed health nutritionist and Revolutionary Beauty Liana Werner-Gray at the back of this book, which will inspire you to begin a lifelong love affair with healthy food.

Creator of *The Earth Diet*, *Cancer-Free Foods*, and *Anxiety-Free with Food*, Liana's mission is to make clean cuisine irresistible. She doesn't skimp on desserts, so you don't have to, either! Find her sunny smile and easy to follow videos on Instagram Stories and YouTube. Liana is a true Revolutionary Beauty! Her amazing culinary creations are preceded by the story of how she healed herself of a golf-ball-size-tumor in her throat through diet, cleansing, and facing emotional issues and traumas that she had never addressed. Both her story and recipes will inspire you!

DaretoDetoxify!

FOOD COMBINING CHART

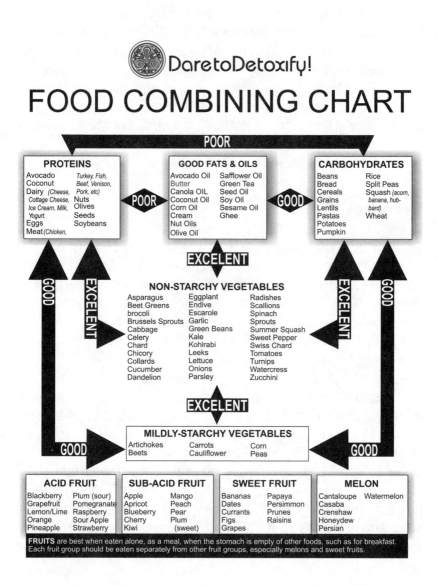

POOR

PROTEINS	
Avocado	Turkey, Fish,
Coconut	Beef, Venison,
Dairy (Cheese,	Pork, etc)
Cottage Cheese,	Nuts
Ice Cream, Milk,	Olives
Yogurt.	Seeds
Eggs	Soybeans
Meat (Chicken,	

POOR

GOOD FATS & OILS	
Avocado Oil	Safflower Oil
Butter	Green Tea
Canola OIL	Seed Oil
Coconut Oil	Soy Oil
Corn Oil	Sesame Oil
Cream	Ghee
Nut Oils	
Olive Oil	

GOOD

CARBOHYDRATES	
Beans	Rice
Bread	Split Peas
Cereals	Squash (acorn,
Grains	banana, hub-
Lentils	bard)
Pastas	Wheat
Potatoes	
Pumpkin	

EXCELENT

NON-STARCHY VEGETABLES

Asparagus	Eggplant	Radishes
Beet Greens	Endive	Scallions
brocoli	Escarole	Spinach
Brussels Sprouts	Garlic	Sprouts
Cabbage	Green Beans	Summer Squash
Celery	Kale	Sweet Pepper
Chard	Kohlrabi	Swiss Chard
Chicory	Leeks	Tomatoes
Collards	Lettuce	Turnips
Cucumber	Onions	Watercress
Dandelion	Parsley	Zucchini

EXCELENT

MILDLY-STARCHY VEGETABLES

Artichokes	Carrots	Corn
Beets	Cauliflower	Peas

(GOOD, EXCELENT, GOOD arrows surround the chart)

ACID FRUIT		SUB-ACID FRUIT		SWEET FRUIT		MELON	
Blackberry	Plum (sour)	Apple	Mango	Bananas	Papaya	Cantaloupe	Watermelon
Grapefruit	Pomegranate	Apricot	Peach	Dates	Persimmon	Casaba	
Lemon/Lime	Raspberry	Blueberry	Pear	Currants	Prunes	Crenshaw	
Orange	Sour Apple	Cherry	Plum	Figs	Raisins	Honeydew	
Pineapple	Strawberry	Kiwi	(sweet)	Grapes		Persian	

FRUITS are best when eaten alone, as a meal, when the stomach is empty of other foods, such as for breakfast. Each fruit group should be eaten separately from other fruit groups, especially melons and sweet fruits.

MODULE 4

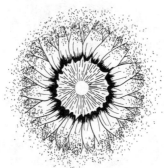

Episode 9
FOOD CRAVINGS &
CANDIDA

"I am on a seafood diet. I see food and I eat it."

—Unkown Author

Food Cravings and Addictions

All dependencies include physiological tentacles, which is why willpower alone is not enough. These tentacles are the toxins from harmful substances.

During a cleanse, we release the toxic residue of these substances, so they no longer hold us hostage. Emancipation becomes effortless. We cease wrestling with the lure of that substance. The body, mind, and spirit are free. This process is akin to releasing a toxic relationship. When we finally muster the courage to walk out the door, we reclaim confidence, optimism, and joy.

Fasting is a powerfully effective tool that supports liberating the body and mind from harmful dependencies. We gain the ability to experience the lightness and clarity of life without toxic substances—or anything else that isn't working. You will be astonished by the emotional and spiritual revelations that appear while fasting.

Candida and Yeast Overgrowth

Do you crave sweets and carbohydrates? Do you experience gas and bloating? Are you fatigued no matter how long you sleep? Do you struggle with brain fog and have trouble concentrating? Does your skin itch or are you prone to rashes?

If you answered "yes" to two or more of these questions, you may suffer from candida—an overgrowth of yeast bacteria. Caused by a high-sugar diet, as well as antibiotic therapy, this common issue often goes unrecognized by conventional medicine. However, candida can be healed through diet, herbs, and, on occasion, medication.

While candida is not life-threatening, this uncomfortable condition can be seriously debilitating and frustrating. Yeast over-growth can cause depression and sap your energy and ability to think. The gut may become gassy and bloated. Who wants to look in the mirror and see a pooched tummy, despite how many sit-ups they do? Anyone who has baked homemade bread knows yeast thrives on sugar. To grow, candida needs food. The insatiable appetite of yeast is a potent source of irrepressible desire for sweets and carbohydrates.

While candida is normally found in the gut, an overgrowth causes gastrointestinal discomfort and disease. Candida can seriously compromise the immune system, disturb your pH balance, and age your skin.

Strange as it may sound, my clients who test positive for candida are usually thrilled! They had been struggling for months or years with symptoms. A positive test signals that their misery is soon to end.

Symptoms that identify a candida overgrowth:

- Headaches
- Skin irritations and rashes
- Bladder or yeast infections
- Gas, bloating, and constipation
- White coating on the tongue (oral thrush)
- Sweet and carb cravings or aversion to protein
- Sinus congestion, allergies, and sinus headaches
- Fatigue, depression, anxiety, concentration issues, and mood swings

You may be living with candida even if you do not experience all these symptoms. For three or more symptoms, we recommend you seek a blood or stool test for candida. Testing kits for vaginal yeast infections are available online or in drug stores. Tests may also indicate systemic candida, particularly if infections are frequent. If prone to candida and yeast infections, scan your home or office for mold. Mold triggers allergies, headaches, chronic sinus infections, and digestive issues—all symptoms of candida.

Stress can activate candida by disturbing the body's pH balance. Therefore, awareness of your emotional state is vital to diagnose and heal yeast overgrowth.

Healing Candida

While doctors often prescribe candida medication, natural herbal formulas work exceedingly well. Most practitioners recommend adhering to candida protocols for 30-60 days. High quality probiotic supplementation promotes and replenishes gut flora.

During treatment for candida overgrowth, desist drinking wine and beer. Refrain from consuming yeast breads, and white flour pastries and pastas. White flour transforms into sugar in your system and feeds candida. Patricia Bragg says, "The whiter the bread, the sooner you're dead!" Die-off symptoms such as fatigue and headaches may arise from candida detoxification. Enemas and colonics provide immense relief from discomfort, while flushing toxins to speed the healing process.

From my experience, diet alone is not enough to heal candida; herbal or naturopathic remedies are required to balance the gut flora. However, diet is crucial in preventing an overgrowth. Below are the *no* and *yes foods* for healing candida. The *no foods* are similar to the *no foods* in "The CARE Fueling Plan."

Candida—No Foods

- Alcohol and beer
- Milk, cheese, and sour cream
- White flour and white flour products
- Foods made with yeast, including whole wheat bread
- Sweeteners with glycemic content, including *healthy **sugar** substitutes* such as honey and agave
- Commercial vinegar, which is different from unfiltered, organic apple cider vinegar (ACV)

Apple cider vinegar (ACV) is made from a yeast added to apple cider, which breaks down the sugar and turns it into alcohol. Then, *good bacteria* is added, turning the alcohol into acetic acid. The resulting ACV appears cloudy, which is active bacteria and highly beneficial for your gut. Called *the mother*, this chunk of cloudy goop in ACV is probiotic—the same good bacteria found in yogurt.

Although ACV generally balances bacteria and flora, it may occasionally activate candida symptoms. Avoid using ACV if you feel it's contributing to a yeast infection or rash. Try freshly squeezed lemon juice on salads rather than any form of vinegar.

Candida—*Yes Foods*

- All fresh vegetables
- Beans, rice, wild rice
- Green vegetable juices
- Nuts, nut butters, and nut milks
- Proteins, including meats and fish
- Gluten-free, yeast-free flatbreads and tortillas
- Cold-pressed olive oil and fresh oils such as avocado

The only fruits that do not feed candida are low-sugar fruits such as grapefruit and berries. For a serious candida over-growth, we recommend no fruit for thirty days.

Fast-Foods Are Not Necessarily Junk Food

"The CARE Fueling Plan" embraces fast-food—just not the ones sold under those familiar golden arches. Below is a list of healthy fast-foods to streamline your life and guard you from reaching for a bag of chips or cookies when not home.

1. Baked sweet potatoes (in portable container)
2. Canned salmon in single portions with zip off lids
3. Edamame, steamed, cooled, and ready to shell and eat
4. Fresh fruit and crispy fresh vegetables, washed, chopped, and kept in ziplock bags
5. Homemade soups or stews in a thermos or to-go cup
6. Hummus with carrots, celery, red and green peppers
7. Nuts and seeds, or nut butters with celery or apples
8. Gluten-free, protein packed muffins
9. Sliced fresh chicken or turkey (no preserved cold cuts)
10. Sugar-free beef jerky or turkey jerky
11. Sugar-free protein bars
12. Sugar-free protein powder in a shaker bottle
13. Superfoods—spirulina, blue-green algae, chlorophyll
14. Vegetable juices, homemade or store-bought, kept in a compact cooler bag or thermos

Succumbing to unhealthy food, wrinkles the skin, and squashes your energy, self-confidence, and self-worth. We have been conditioned to use food as comfort—to numb sadness and anger. You may feel these emotions more acutely as you detoxify. Remember that *feeling* reminds us we are alive and capable of change. Overnight successes do not actually happen overnight. Shifting how we fuel ourselves is a step-by-step process. That is the pay-off for years spent on this planet. Revolutionary Beauties see the cycles of life, with respect for each. This new journey represents a birth cycle—and birth is beautiful, messy, and infinitely rewarding.

"The CARE Fueling Plan" provides tools to sugar and junk proof your choices. You may find your beloved lemon pie is even more delicious as a birthday treat than as a daily diversion. You may discover that feeling clearheaded and full of energy is a gift too precious to surrender—even on holidays. Once in charge, your choices become more clear.

Slow Down to Speed Up

How would you like to come home to fresh, hot, hearty meals ready and waiting? I'm not talking about hiring a personal chef. Enter the slow cooker or Crock Pot! They are back in style and for good reason. These inexpensive purveyors of delicious food are not just for facilitating fast, easy dinners. They allow the busiest people to wake up to hot curry or chicken stew, ready to pour into a lunch thermos.

The internet is teeming with recipes for healthy slow cooked lunches and dinners. Make your recipe as simple as filling the pot with veggies, broth, and half an organic chicken and herbs. Experiment with ethnic foods that adapt well to slow cooking, to offer tenderized meats and exotic vegan or vegetarian cuisine. I lean toward simple recipes. You may adore the creativity of complex gourmet meals. Whatever your skill level, slow cooking makes anyone into a chef. Slow cooking is one of my favorite fast ways to enjoy healthy food.

I Know What to Do, I Just Can't Do it

That is the single most common sentence uttered in my clinic over 40 years. Who can't relate? As we begin the health journey, the recurrent mental picture of that coveted comfort food sends the most stouthearted soul straight to the nearest bakery or pizza parlor!

"The CARE Toolbox" incorporates food enzymes, which are key in weight loss and weight maintenance. They reduce that muffin top, as well as cellulite. "The CARE Fueling Plan" is designed to kick your metabolism into high gear. The weight will, little by little, dissolve.

Tools for Cravings

- For intense cravings—Seek a blood or stool test for candida. Treat, if necessary, with herbs and diet.
- Candida Detoxification Protocol—Eliminate uncomfortable symptoms with saunas, steams, salt baths, dry skin brushing, and colonics. Kick those toxins down the road! Toxins are a major source of cravings.
- Fill up with protein—Digestible protein is the number one antidote to sugar and carb cravings! Protein shakes are my secret weapon. I never leave home without one. Because protein powder does not require refrigeration, it travels well. Add sugar-free liquid of choice—from water to almond milk, then shake. This form of liquid protein is a lifesaver for kids and parents. When blood sugar crashes, even the strongest can't keep from going over the edge!
- Hydrate, hydrate, hydrate—Dehydration mimics blood sugar crashes. When craving a pick-me-up, sip eight ounces of electrolyte water. This may clear your head and reboot your energy immediately.

Patricia Bragg enjoys two scoops of Vanilla All Day Energy in her morning shake. I developed this protein powder during my decades-long search for healthy, portable nutrition. This delicious sugar, gluten, and dairy-free blend are sweetened with monk fruit powder—which has no aftertaste.

Breakfast Versus "The No Breakfast Plan"

If imbibing in breakfast, try lighter options such as:

- Herbal tea and organic bone broth
- Fresh vegetable juice (no high-sugar fruit juice)
- Protein shake with water and ice; add spinach, kale, a slice of apple, pear, or frozen berries for sweetness

Or, if breakfast is your jam, try these healthy alternatives to intermittent fasting or the "No Breakfast Plan:"

- Tofu scramble with vegetables
- Hormone-free organic sausages
- Organic avocado toast on spelt bread
- Seed cheese or goat cheese with fresh fruit
- Gluten-free, sugar-free muffin with butter or ghee
- Nut or seed butter of choice with banana, apple slices, or on a rice cake
- Oatmeal sweetened with monk fruit, agave, or a dab of honey
- Organic eggs any style, without cheese (unless goat cheese)

Lunch Suggestions

Aside from Dr. Mark Hyman's favorite—a can of sardines over a salad—fast, affordable, and high protein lunches include:

- Pureed vegetable soup
- Slow cooked bean soup, chili, or curry
- Canned wild caught salmon with salad

- Gluten-free pasta with olive oil and veggies
- Broiled fish, chicken, or tofu, with veggies or salad
- Protein shake with almond butter and frozen fruit
- *The Big Salad* with a hard-boiled or soft poached egg and lots of veggies
- Baked sweet potato with butter or ghee, even if previously baked and eaten cold or warm
- Fresh roasted turkey slices (no cold cuts) and avocado

Dinner in Ten

See Patricia Bragg's "10 Minute Tuesday" recipes on Facebook and Instagram for delicious, healthy entrees ready in 10 minutes and great for any day of the week! Or, double slow cooker and other recipes from the previous episode to allow next day 10-minute lunches and snacks.

1. Try these recipes posted on Patricia's social media and website, patricabragg.com.

    - 10-Minute *Caprese* Salad
    - 10-Minute Glazed Salmon
    - 10-Minute Chickpea Tapas
    - 10-Minute Dilled Egg Salad
    - 10-Minute Miso-Tofu Salad
    - 10-Minute Miso Ramen Soup
    - 10-Minute Black Bean Scramble
    - 10-Minute Gluten-free Pesto Pasta
    - 10-Minute Beet and Goat Cheese Salad
    - 10-Minute Fried Rice with Stir-Fried Vegetables

2. Practice "The CARE Fueling Plan" daily and your body will love you—and you will love your body!
3. Be patient as your body changes—and it will. Give yourself three months to truly change your eating habits. And, trust that in nine months, these habits will be second nature. You will be stronger, brighter, and happier than you are now—maybe than you've

ever been. Furthermore, you will enjoy consistent moods and the ability to rescue yourself from food cravings and binge eating. You will see yourself in the mirror and be amazed at your sparkle.

Exercises

1. Breathe—When you need to draw strength, be with nature. Breathe and ask for guidance. Mother Nature never fails to deliver. She is, like you, powerful beyond measure. Practice breathing techniques from "Module 1." Breathing in and out slowly to the count of seven, three times until calm, will disconnect you from *fight or flight* and bring you back to the present. Food cravings are often accompanied by feelings of panic. You can do this!
2. Move Your Body—Go for a brisk walk, jump on the rebounder, and stretch for 20 minutes.
3. Connect—Call a friend or write in your journal.
4. Create—Paint, draw, write a poem or prayer, and remember, creativity fills the soul.
5. Fast—Fasting and intermittent fasting permanently relieve cravings, especially when accompanied by detoxification protocols and drinking pure water.

MODULE 5

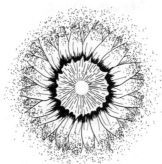

Episode 10
MOVEMENT & EXERCISE

"If you want to live, move!"
—Elaine LaLanne, *First Lady of Fitness*

Patricia Bragg represents the gold standard for fitness and longevity. In March 2020, Elaine LaLanne—widow of Jack LaLanne (Paul Bragg's most famous protégé)—inducted Patricia into the National Fitness Hall of Fame. Patricia's fiery proclamation, "You have 640 muscles in your body and you must use them or lose them," reached worldwide audiences. She motivated millions of Bragg followers to "stop living by calendar years, get off the couch, touch their toes, stand up straight, and reach for the stars!"

In Patricia's youth, exercise was widely viewed as inappropriate for women—other than housework, of course! America sampled their first taste of fitness watching Patricia and her father work out on their 1950s television show. This dynamic duo led the first outdoor exercise classes on the beach in Waikiki, Hawaii. Although half their size, Patricia never imagined herself less capable than men. No one would catch this whirling dervish cleaning the bathroom—she was outside playing tennis!

Inspired by Patricia's lust for fitness, another famous Bragg protégé, Jane Fonda, made "going for the burn" not only suitable for women, but desirable. Jane Fonda made aerobics sexy and popular with her iconic 1980s home video series, "Jane Fonda's Workout." Through her, women learned to exercise at home, lose weight, and feel great in their bodies. Thanks to these trailblazers, we have shamelessly been dancing, kicking, stretching, and jogging away stress ever since. According to Patricia Bragg, the key to ageless beauty and vitality is to never stop moving!

Hormone and immune health is directly linked to daily exercise—as are energy level and mood. Movement pumps heart rate—a critical piece of the longevity puzzle. This is crucial, as heart disease is a leading cause of death for women in the United States. Like flossing, we know we should exercise.

What if you would rather watch a movie than twist yourself into a pretzel? What if you consider running till you are a puddle of perspiration, unattractive and uninteresting?

If your answers are "yes," this module was made for you. Creating Ageless Renewable Energy (CARE) does not require countless hours in the gym. In the privacy of your home, through basic and timeless techniques, "The CARE Movement and Fitness Plan" is designed to reduce inflammation. These tools allow you to earn limber, sinewy muscles, and strong bones—while reintroducing your body to the playfulness and joy of easy movement.

As we embrace the three keys of fitness—flexibility, stamina, and strength—we liberate ourselves from false, paralyzing ideals of perfection and competition. We prioritize fun, which keeps us moving—and smiling.

As Paul Bragg and Patricia Bragg wrote, "We recommend that you see your doctor or health practitioner before starting our practice ... and again in one year, so they can document the transformation that the Bragg Healthy Lifestyle offers!" Nothing builds morale and self-confidence like improvement—especially the kind we are conditioned to believe is impossible after 40, 60, or even 80! During her speech honoring Patricia, Elaine LaLanne left the audience laughing and clapping when she could still drop to the floor and "do 20" push-ups when she was 91!

Changing Beliefs, Transforming Bodies

Recently, I watched a video featuring a 75-year-old body worker project herself from a cross-legged position on the floor, to standing tall—in one, elegant swoop. That simple act took my breath away. Her effortless movements showed me what is possible for the body, at any age—which elicited questions I asked myself:

- What do I believe my body is capable of right now?
- What might I gain from having a flexible, strong, pain-free body?
- Am I willing to release previous perceptions and beliefs about my body, and embrace a new vision of radical aliveness?

Ask yourself these same questions, without censoring the response. When is the last time you felt fit? You may feel that reclaiming your body's ability to move effortlessly is overwhelming. This may seem like a nose-to-the-grindstone process, akin to doing taxes! You might even have purchased gym memberships or exercise equipment that went unused. Most of us, including me, have done the same.

As a Revolutionary Beauty, your exercise history is irrelevant. We are starting anew, today, to build a beautiful body that carries you gracefully. We do this because a lithe body not only feels fabulous, but also connects us to sensuality and creativity. Flexibility, stamina, and strength liberate bodies and spirits. This expands horizons of possibilities in life. When achy, stiff, and swollen, we easily imagine our best years are over. As we know, discipline alone does not demolish old belief systems. We must carve new neuro pathways in the brain that welcome a new vision of ourselves.

CARE Movement Blueprint

To create a blueprint of your new physique, write a story about a time when you felt light and easy in your body. Recall when you were engaged so fully that you felt as if your body did not exist. Maybe you were a child running across a field, skating, flying high on the swings at school, or practicing yoga in college. This may be a moment on vacation when you swam with dolphins or played beach volleyball with reckless abandon. Describe how you felt, what you saw, smelled, tasted, and touched with as much detail as possible.

- What does this freedom in your body feel like and look like?
- How does this ease of movement affect your self-worth?
- How does this story inform your vision about what life will be like in five or ten years?
- How is this visualization different from the way you feel right now?

Your story will reconnect you to trust your body's capabilities, and how natural that physical flow can feel.

Now, as you did in "Module 1," create a second story about your future self, who rises in the morning, stretches like a cat, and strides to the kitchen with a bounce in her step. As you dress, notice the muscular definition in your arms and legs. This future self looks and feels decades younger, stands tall, and moves with confidence.

Let's Get Moving

If you already enjoy a fitness ritual, you're ahead of the game. Keep doing it! However, if you are not drawn to fitness, the most fun and effective way to launch into a routine is with the companionship of a *fitness buddy*. Your fitness buddy is a friend, partner, or colleague who keeps you accountable and meets you for early morning walks, sunset hikes, or in-home dance parties. Especially at the start of a movement program—when we need motivation—fitness buddies are invaluable.

Where to begin? Start walking. Research has shown that 30 minutes a day of brisk walking, 4-5 days a week, is as effective for cardiovascular health as running or jogging. This form of exercise is easy on the hips and knees.

Patricia Bragg's testimony to walking is, "Walking brings more of the body into healthy action than anything else!"

Arianna Huffington, creator of the Huffington Post, reports that she no longer takes meetings sitting down. Earbuds in place, she creates, brainstorms, and manages her staff while hiking in the hills near her office. Nationally known child sleep expert, Dr. Angelique Millette, does walking consultations with moms and their babies—a serene respite in nature for everyone. A dozen of my clients take meetings while moving, thanks to remote working. Research has shown that many of us think better on our feet.

Who says you need to sit behind a desk to be productive? Revolutionary Beauties create a unique, exciting new world. Let's design one that works for bodies and minds.

If your neighborhood is not conducive to walking, treadmills are now more affordable than a new computer. My favorite form of exercise is running on an elliptical machine, designed to take stress from joints and limbs. I fell in love with my husband's elliptical machine when we married. Convenience is key, and elliptical machines can be adjusted for any level of activity. Thirty minutes fly by quickly. When I began, rehabilitating a broken ankle, I could only handle 15 minutes at a time. In three months, I built strength and stamina. So can you.

Do you love to dance, but can't find time to attend dance classes? Hundreds of choices are at our fingertips online— jazz, ballet, modern. Many are free. *Santa Barbara's Zumba Queen*, Josette Tkacik, one of the world's most successful Zumba instructors, has duplicated the energy, passion, and inspiration of her in person classes with online streaming. Consider something completely new—belly dancing, pole dancing, tap dancing—take a leap. Do something you've always wanted to try. No one is watching. No one is judging.

The internet offers an infinite feast of online fitness classes:

- Pilates
- Yoga
- Weight lifting
- Stretching
- Tai Chi
- Aikido
- Kung Fu

I have asked experts in each of these categories to share their favorite online classes and teachers. Find them in the Resource Guide at the back of this book.

Though she loved all sports, Patricia adored tennis. She was on the court as often as possible well into her seventies. She also loved dancing, swimming, and gardening, which she said was a spiritual experience that connected her to all living beings. One client, Suzanne, recently took up horseback riding at 65. She had always wanted to ride horses, but never could. This was her gift to herself for years of hard work.

Suzanne says: "I grew up watching movies of beautiful girls galloping horseback across the plains. Well, I grew up in New York City. Only wealthy girls had horses and riding lessons in Central Park. I promised myself that after college, I would move to the country, and get a horse. Instead, I got a job in another big city and life just took off. There was never the time or money, but I would dream of horses, the way I did as a kid. I felt so foolish!

Then, one day, it just hit me: *If not now, when?* I found a barn that offered riding lessons, dipped into my savings, and started riding. At first, I was frightened—horses are big! I'm no kid anymore, and I was out of shape. People think riding means just sitting on a horse's back with the horse doing all the work, but it's a workout! Every muscle was sore. But, all I can say is that it's like falling in love, the feeling I had—the smell of the horse's breath, the excitement of being on his back. I can't wait to go to the barn and saddle him up. It's the high point of my week. You know, I think this horse saved my life."

Marie, a 66-year-old paralegal, enrolled in belly dancing classes and shared that she unexpectedly "feels like a teenager again. I feel so free! It makes me cry to tell you that I'd lost that part of myself, while caring for my husband, who's been ill, and working long hours to get my kids through college. My daughter said to me the other day, 'What are you doing, mom? You're so happy!' I told her, it's the dancing. I just love it. Who knew? I never weigh myself, but I was at the doctor last week, and discovered that I had lost ten pounds!"

Another client shares this story of beginning a yoga practice. "I was beginning to walk like 'an old person,' I joked to Margie, my best friend, meaning, I felt stiffer every day—all over! I told her, 'At this rate, I'll be crawling in five years—if I'm lucky!' My back was killing me. She said, 'Well, come to yoga class with me.' That scared the heck out of me, the idea of everyone watching me struggle to touch my toes. I used to be an athlete, so this state of affairs was particularly depressing.

Anyway, she said that her instructor had video classes, and she would come over and do them with me in my home. We started—me, slow as molasses. But, believe it or not, in six months, I'm no yogi, but I stopped needing weekly visits to the chiropractor. My back is so much better! I have more energy, and sleep like a baby. It's amazing. I wish I'd started years ago. I tell everyone, it's never too late."

The goal is to find something you love, a form of movement so compelling that to practice four days a week is easy. Pin the mindset story of your future self in your closet, mirror, or desk as inspiration. Grab a fitness buddy, or fly solo. Protect this precious time as you would an appointment with a technical expert with whom you've waited for weeks to see!

Beginning is the Hardest Part

Even fitness lovers Paul Bragg and Patricia Bragg knew that the first ten minutes of exercise is the hardest part.

In the Bragg Healthy Lifestyle, the Braggs write: "The successful student of the Bragg Healthy Lifestyle, and anyone who has successfully made healthy exercise part of their daily routine, will tell you the same thing. The moment of beginning is the most difficult. The moment before you put that one leg in front of the other on the first step of your brisk walk is the most difficult moment of exercise."

The people who tell the success stories of exercise recommend playing the *ten-minute-trick*. Before you start, tell yourself, I'm only going to do this—walk, jog, bounce—for ten minutes, and then I'll stop. Once you've done that, you will likely surprise yourself when you realize those ten minutes were over ten minutes ago. And you had fun! Now you are on the path to healthy fitness.

Flexibility, Stamina, and Strength

Below are forms of exercise to support fitness categories:

Flexibility:
- Golf
- Yoga
- Pilates
- Stretching
- Martial arts
- Dance classes
- Tennis
- Bowling
- Swimming
- Table tennis
- Equestrian sports

Stamina:
- Hiking
- Cycling
- Peloton
- Jogging
- Running
- Elliptical
- Treadmill
- Fast walking
- Weight lifting
- Cardio and aerobics
- Dance
- Tennis
- Walking
- Volleyball
- Gardening
- Swimming
- Rebounder
- Martial arts
- Racquetball
- Equestrian sports

Strength and Balance:
- Yoga
- Pilates
- Gardening
- Martial arts
- Rock climbing
- Lifting weights
- Kayaking
- Rebounder
- Pool therapy
- Physical therapy
- Resistance stretching
- Stand up paddle board

Some forms of exercise are one-stop-shopping practices, as they embrace the three foundational fitness components. Yet, if your regular routine is brisk walking, the flexibility aspect needs to be addressed. Ask yourself, is my chosen fitness ritual targeting flexibility, stamina, and strength or balance? If not, how can I augment my practice?

As women, we need to pay particular attention to building bone density. One method is to lift light weights when we walk or watch television or a movie. If you've wondered how Michelle Obama earned those beautifully sculpted arms, she reports that she lifts weights daily, for both her strength and sanity. My client, Lina recently wore a lovely summer sheath to her son's wedding. She shared that "after seeing a picture of the skin under my arms flapping in the wind like a pelican, I went out and bought weights immediately!" Lina is an avid hiker, but hiking does little to tone arms.

Rebounding is a fantastic form of exercise. Revolutionary Beauty Goldie Hawn recently posted a video on social media of herself bouncing on a rebounder, while doing arm circles, with music blasting. I noticed that she was only bouncing a few inches into the air. High jumps are unnecessary when rebounding. Excellent for core strength, building gorgeous tushies, and stamina, rebounding is a lot of fun. Small rebounders easily fit into the corner of an office or living room.

Just Do it!

For some, only a national emergency would cause them to break an appointment to walk, run, play tennis, or attend yoga class. Whether a relief from stress, anxiety, or for the joy of sliding into jeans, this group experiences a bliss that compels commitment.

What if you have never felt that bliss? Like healthy eating habits, fasting, and cleansing, the reward is substantial. If you commit to a fitness ritual for at least 30 minutes, four times a week for three months, you will be hooked. The payoff? You will look and feel like a whole new person. You can do this.

Draw on the muscle memory you have built for *doing hard things*. If you're reading this book, you have consistently *shown up* for something, or someone—whether you wanted to or not. That's what Revolutionary Beauties do—even if sometimes to our detriment. The silver lining is, through adversity, we have earned authenticity. As Glennon Doyle said in her best seller, *Untamed,* "We can do hard things." We now commit the time and energy that we spent on others to "The CARE Fitness Plan." This plan exudes the power to renew spirits and reconnect us to our bodies.

Action Steps

The CARE Fitness Plan

1. Create your body blueprint meditation—remember the future body you had envisioned in your writing at the beginning of this episode.
2. See your doctor for any issues or previous injuries, and if any issues arise, enlist the professional support of a physical therapist, trainer, or fitness specialist.
3. Commit to 30 minutes of exercise per day, four days per week, for three months—starting light and easy, and build as you like.
4. Find a fitness buddy for accountability and support.
5. If you need alone time, structure your fitness routine so that you are uninterrupted.
6. Try something new! Experiment with different forms of exercise until you find something you love.
7. Talk to yourself for support and encouragement, as you would a child learning to ride a bike. Use positive affirmations rather than allowing negative self-talk to overwhelm and discourage you. Motivational audio tapes can be helpful.
8. Stay hydrated. Boost your hydration with electrolytes during workouts. Reach for healthy snacks such as protein shakes or digestible snacks—not sugar or carbs.
9. Reward yourself weekly with a massage, salt bath, sauna, and yes—even a bit of dark chocolate (preferably sugar-free) for working out.
10. Take before and after pictures to measure progress.

Revolutionary Beauty Josette Tkacik

Josette is Zumba Fitness' most successful instructor, a wife, mother, and professional dancer who healed herself natural- ly of life-threatening, "incurable" rheumatoid arthritis. She is passionately committed to sharing her story, tools, insights, and courses. You can find her on Zoom daily. She welcomes all ages and abilities, including those with disabilities that previously never felt comfortable on a dance floor.

I asked her, "how did you get to where you are now from suffering such a debilitating disease?"

Josette: *I did not start out healthy, not by a long shot, so that would really be my starting point—the day I lost my health to disease.*

It's very easy to not think about the deeper levels of health, body function, mind-body-soul awareness when everything is going great. But when you are too late, and disease hits, you are forced onto a path that takes your journey into what I call ... magic.

I lost my health, my world, and the floor beneath me in Febru- ary of 2011. Ultimately, the excruciating pain, inability to move, and the feeling of deep "malaise" was diagnosed as advanced rheumatoid arthritis, an autoimmune disease categorized as "incurable." The best doctors hoped to accomplish is to put the patient in "remission."

RA, as it is referred to, is unbearably painful. I would have gladly gone through childbirth a hundred times over than go through a week of RA. As your body starts to destroy itself, by essentially deconstructing your joints, it's like having ev- ery joint at one time or another in your body break, tweak, or otherwise, be destroyed. Holding my two-year-old was nearly impossible, and the emotional pain that it caused became the catalyst for my journey.

I think, myself, like most people, want a quick fix. But western medicine's protocol is a lifetime of toxic meds with side effects comparable to the disease itself. The best that the meds can do is allow you to function. But it is no cure and the damage the pills and shots do to your body are a huge price to pay. Quick fixes are an illusion. They don't hold water. A lifetime of meds isn't sustainable.

Before I got sick, I was living with incredible stress. It was right after the 2008 crash and my husband lost his job. Financially, we were broke. We had an amazing baby who was and is "our everything." But, at that time, before RA, my husband and I fought so much that we eventually separated. The stress, angst, and misery were so severe that I distinctly remember sobbing one day and saying to myself, "This can't be good for me!" My whole body had such deep grief and sorrow. I thought, "I hope I don't get sick."

Stress lowers your immune system. And I was no exception. Two months before I was diagnosed with RA, late 2010, I got walking pneumonia. Doctors put me on a long list of antibiotics; in fact, I had to go into the hospital so they could administer them (the antibiotics) intravenously. In retrospect, the toll that stress and my lifestyle had taken on my body was manifesting into illness. I just wasn't listening. I kept hitting the override button. I left my body in the hands of western medicine and kept on with my toxic lifestyle. I was sad, fighting with my husband, angry, and not caring too much about the deeper message my body was trying to send me. Of course, doctors don't tell you that stress, diet, and lifestyle are the root cause of illness. Two months of antibiotics for walking pneumonia and RA entered my life. On that day, everything stopped.

When you cannot move, and are in bone-breaking pain 100 percent of the time, it gets your attention, and your focus. **Now**, *I was paying attention. But was it too late?*

"You have rheumatoid arthritis and fibromyalgia. Looks like you have major joint damage already."

That doctor quickly wrote a prescription for methotrexate, (a chemotherapy drug); prednisone (a steroid), and a biologic, aimed at completely shutting down my immune system—so don't catch a cold, you may die.

"You're going to have to take these for the rest of your life."

But wait! *How did I get here? What is causing this? How can I heal? This **cannot** happen to me. I am a mom! I am a dancer. And, those questions, along with the arrogant and evasive nonresponse from so-called experts began the most wonderful journey of my life.*

There was one light—one beautiful light beckoning in the darkness—it was consistent and it had my heart. That light was my two-year-old son, Tomas. I kept looking at him, and a powerful, passionate voice inside my head would say, "Josette, you have to figure this out, because we're more than this!"

But where to start?

I began my digging for information with endless internet searches. I began to slowly put the puzzle pieces together.

The first thing I began to understand is I needed to start with three things—my gut, my alkalinity, and my lifestyle.

I realized having just had five rounds of antibiotics for pneumonia, that it would be food for a yeast overgrowth and, in fact, ultimately systemic candida. Candida can cause perforations in the gut lining causing leaky gut, which in turn causes an immune response.

I wondered immediately why didn't any of the doctors tell me this? I found this widely prevalent on holistic and integrative websites that sincerely seemed interested in helping people understand disease and healing. But it was nowhere in western medicine—nowhere.

So, I began the process of healing my gut, which first meant eliminating systemic candida. I understood from my research that this was not an overnight task. It would involve candida die-off and eliminating toxins.

Thank goodness I learned before—or else I would not have survived the journey.

The key ingredient for healing systemic candida was organic ACV! That was huge for me. ACV alkalizes your body, which is was a huge issue in disease and candida. Disease rarely exists in an alkaline environment and candida simply cannot survive it. Alkalizing was the path to healing—it was vital. So here I am. In complete physical pain from RA, refusing meds and trying to be a mom with very limited ability—trying to piece a puzzle together that was overwhelming.

At the time I was living in Florida, but my heart longed to be back in Santa Barbara, where I had lived for 20 years before moving to follow my husband's career. I looked daily for want ads to maybe find a way back, and then—there it was. The City of Santa Barbara was looking for a Zumba instructor. I had gotten my license to teach a month earlier as fate would have it, right before disease hit.

I flew to Santa Barbara and had a friend help me into the elevator to interview for the Zumba Instructor position. I gave my best Academy Award winning performance of utter wellness (while in excruciating pain). My interview was five minutes long. My friend waited at the bottom of the elevator for me to exit to help me back into the car.

I got the job!

By that time, I had already shifted my diet, but I was still in incredible pain. I was trying to navigate the various flares, inflammation, and unbelievable pain while caring for my two-year-old and now, moving to my beloved Santa Barbara.

Family and friends were no support. After all, I was not mobile, partially disabled, sitting on the heels of a diagnosis of going into a wheelchair, and making the announcement that I am moving to California to teach Zumba. It was received as irresponsible and chaotic. No one understood why I didn't just do as the doctors told me to do.

That was the moment I finally learned a lesson that came to me over and over in the past, but I had never realized how important until that second. Follow your heart no matter what.

I financed my move by selling an antique gold necklace that I had received from my grandmother, who had received it from her grandmother. This one piece of jewelry that landed in my hands was worth several thousands—just enough for three months rent in Santa Barbara.

I sold it. Everyone thought I was insane.

When I took my job, I was still in pain, but I was a little better. My healing was, as most people's is, two steps forward and one step back. There were days when a healing crisis would have me feeling like I had the flu. But, I always showed up to teach my Zumba class and I always showed up for my son. There was an emotional healing as well that happened simultaneously. I flat out told my husband, "I love you and I don't want to fight anymore. My goal is to show up for my son and be his superhero."

My husband joined me in Santa Barbara three weeks later and said, "I'm here to support you one hundred percent." He delivered newspapers the first year so he could earn some money and we barely survived—but what an adventure.

With RA, the mornings are the worst—just to give an idea of how unable to move I was, if I woke in the middle of the night to go to the bathroom, I had to wake my husband so he could carry me there.

Little by little by little, step by step. Two steps forward one step back.

My diet consisted of alkaline foods, a lot of juicing, smoothies, and greens, greens, greens. I was like a rabbit. I ate raw, vegan—and tested my urine acid daily to get an idea of how I was doing. I could feel my body getting healthy. I saw the dead candida coming out of my body in my feces. I knew all that I was doing was effective. And, I continued—the pain was ever present though, albeit a little better.

When I began teaching, I had three students. I could barely move, to be transparent, I did take ibuprofen before class. I would dig deep, because I thought, if I don't make this work, how will I feed my son? The City was just about to pull the plug on the class, and I had to get myself in gear and show up like I never had before, every single day.

Michael Bernard Beckwith says, "Pain pushes until a vision pulls." This is where I was—the pain pushed me towards my vision of a better life—a life without disease.

I never said anything to anyone about my RA; I was afraid of losing my job. But, in retrospect teaching Zumba was catalyst to my healing, because there was a freedom, mindset, shift in my consciousness that happened in that class—a connection with Source. I was able to shift from fear to hope to complete wellness inside my soul. That feeling and knowing just reflected in my physical.

I had to transcend my physical vessel because my body was in so much pain. I learned and understood deeply that I was not my body. I was my spirit, and even though we're in class to move, feel our flexibility and our strength, and develop our core, the intent is always about loving our bodies and connecting to our spirit. Bodies change all the time! To me, it seems one-dimensional to say, "I want my body to look a certain way, because then I'll be happy." The intent of my class is to give everyone permission to embrace our bodies as they are, and see them as beautiful, in all the different shapes and sizes while drinking from a deeper well, so to speak. My class transcends the body, just as I had to.

There's so much power inside of us. That's my greatest message, that connecting to that, to Source, to ourselves makes anything possible. It's not like you do it once and get a diploma, you commit to it every day. The soul can do so much more than the body, and the body follows the heart.

Within a year I was completely symptom free and began to live the unimaginable life.

In 2016, a doctor who attends my class asked to take my blood work. I told her, I did not need to know—I felt healthier than ever, but she insisted—more because she wanted to see how my RA numbers were. My blood work came back completely disease free. No RA, no sign of any disease, which of course, as far as western medicine is concerned, is impossible.

I was declared a scientific medical miracle. A name given when doctors cannot explain it. But, I knew how I healed. And, I had a deep understanding that we all have the intrinsic power to heal. Today, I told my son, now 12, "Don't ever try to fit in—let your heart lead." And he said, "I'm not, I'm going to create my own extraordinary life!"

So, this is the legacy I have the privilege of leaving for my son and I will not stop voicing our power. My journey is a gift, because now I have the operator's manual. Now, I can be the resource for someone else. Life is beautiful.

Josette's Practice for Your Soul

Movement can be a meditation. Movement can align you with your deeper being. Movement should always be authentic and not contrived as an expression. Here is Josette's practice to help create authentic movement.

1. Call all your energy back. Whether we know it or not, we can lose fragments of our sovereign power down the timeline of our lives, and indeed in past lives. Traumas, thoughts about what happened yesterday, last year or tomorrow contribute to this fragmented energy. I like to do this practice to open any sacred movement. Intention is enough, but be clear, "I call all my energy and attention back to this now moment from every place, time, and reality."

2. Music is the language of the soul. Find music that resonates with you. If it doesn't excite you, or literally **move** you, don't play it for this exercise. I have created a playlist that I love.

3. Authentic movement. The first step in movement is start moving your feet, side to side. Step, tap, step, tap. See how the rest of your body wants to flow with the music. Some may find that their arms take flight, others find that their direction shifts. Listen to the authenticity of your heart as it connects to the music— and flow. Allow your feet to guide you body.

4. Awareness of your heart space. During this practice keep returning your attention to your heart. Stay there. Listen. Allow yourself to create this space—a sacred space for your heart to release, express, and shine. If tears flow, allow them. If laughter ensues cherish it. There is no wrongdoing here.

Find Josette's music for dancing and fitness on her website listed in the Resource Guide.

MODULE 5

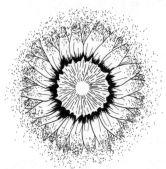

Episode 11
YOGA & PILATES

"Whenever we have stiffness in the body, our mind should be especially supple. It is never the stiffness in our body that limits our practice, it is always the stiffness of our mind."

—Geeta Iyengar, Codirector of the
Ramamani Iyengar Memorial Yoga Institute and
Author of *Yoga: A Gem for Women*

No chapter on movement would be complete without acknowledging yoga as one of the founding pillars of fitness. Birthed in India as a spiritual practice, this ancient tradition is now in the spotlight it has always deserved. Yoga centers now abound in nearly every city in America.

In my early twenties, a friend dragged me to an afternoon class at the original Bikram hot yoga studio in Beverly Hills. Within a week, I was hooked. The ninety minutes a day I spent strengthening and stretching every muscle, and building core power changed the shape of my body. Yoga transformed how I felt when I looked in the mirror and the way I carried myself. Each class left me feeling exhilarated and cleansed.

However, my joyful days at the studio ended when, after class, Bikram tried to kiss me, as I attempted to escape into my car. Although many great teachers are flawed, nothing could take away what yoga poured into my soul. To see my son, Luke, lead a yoga class on the beach is to witness the authenticity and enduring wisdom of a 5,000-year-old ritual.

In addition to stretching, strengthening, and promoting balance, research shows that yoga can also:

- Improve sleep
- Relieve chronic pain
- Relieve inflammation
- Help people quit smoking
- Strengthen the immune system
- Relieve symptoms of menopause
- Aids the elimination of addictions
- Reduce anxiety, stress, and depression
- Boost metabolism and support weight loss

One of yoga's finest attributes is that anyone can practice anywhere, anytime. No equipment needed! Yoga can be adjusted to your fitness level and done on your schedule.

- Yoga is offered in many styles
- Kundalini is based on energy movement
- Iyenger is comprised of precise movements
- Restorative yoga is calm and relaxed, and focuses on breath and stress release
- For those seeking an active, athletic practice, consider Vinyasa and Ashtanga

My dear friend, Cheri Clampett, created Therapeutic Yoga (therapeuticyoga.com) for those who desire a gentle, yet effective practice. Her specialty is to assist cancer and trauma survivors, and those with limited mobility. She facilitates them to achieve balance, and to feel safe and whole again after surgery or a life changing event. Her students feel a restored sense of self and well-being they thought they would never reclaim. See the Resource Guide for a variety of online classes, and enjoy yoga at home.

Many classes are free! Start slow and don't push. Overdoing causes pulled muscles. The term, *no pain, no gain*, may apply to some aspects of life, but not to most physical activities. Pain frequently translates into *paying for it later!* Pay attention to your body. Slow the breath. Be present. Watch your body transform as the mind calms and thinking clears.

Revolutionary Beauty Cheri Clampett

Meet Cheri Clampett. Cheri is a certified yoga therapist with over 25 years experience teaching yoga. She has presented Therapeutic Yoga, which she founded, at Beth Israel Medical Center and Langone Medical Center in New York City, and is the coauthor of *Therapeutic Yoga Kit*.

Therapeutic Yoga is a particularly effective practice for those recovering from, or living with, trauma, injury, or illness. This practice combines restorative yoga, breathwork, hands-on healing, and guided meditation techniques in such a way that is gentle, yet effective for bringing the body into balance and reducing stress. Soft-spoken and beautiful, Cheri looks the same as when I first met her 30 years ago.

Julia: Who is your inspiration for health and beauty?

Cheri: *Laura Huxley. She had a huge influence on me, and taught me how differently we age when we move and do yoga. Talk about sexy and beautiful, she was all that and more in her nineties! She was my mentor for 23 years.*

Julia: And how did you discover yoga?

Cheri: *I was taken by friends, rather reluctantly, to a yoga class in my twenties. At the end of class I had a sense that something*

was very wrong with my body. Shortly afterward, I was diagnosed with cancer and had surgery; this was in my late twenties. And, the powerful awareness I had that day never left me.
I thought about it, time and time again, lying in stillness at the
end of class, having this knowing, this moment of tuning into
myself, and it changed my life. It changed my whole direction.

I became passionate about the question, how do we heal? How
do we have a deeper connection with our body?

It's been a lifelong journey. I had a recurrence of cancer, and
that led me to a recognition of childhood trauma. That's
when I did the deeper emotional work, and the energy work.
I explored the connection between health, the mind, and the
body. And, I learned about healing through food, and now, I
am totally plant based. Meeting the body, with all its different
needs affects our energy, and how we heal.

As I was healing, I became so passionate about yoga. I took
yoga classes, but even though I loved it, I was so shy that I
didn't think I would ever actually teach. I studied massage and
energy healing, and trained to become a yoga teacher, but I
thought I would only do private sessions.

After I finished that training, I would go take a yoga class, and
somebody would say, "Oh, the teacher can't make it, why don't
you teach the class?" This happened over and over again, and I
decided that I just had to get out of my own way and do it! The
Universe kind of pushed me into it. I recognized there was such
a need. This was during the AIDS crisis in Los Angeles before
the antiviral drugs were available, and so many of my friends
were dying. I started offering free classes to people with HIV
and AIDS.

Anna Delury, a protege of Geeta Iyengar, was my teacher at
the time. She gave me the first taste of restorative yoga, although back then, it was mostly taught in prenatal classes.
I thought, this is great for anyone who is healing. It was so

mindful, so gentle, and yet, I felt so wonderful afterwards. By the way, Anna is still teaching. So, I started to bring restorative yoga to my classes for people with HIV and AIDS. For those asymptomatic and healthy, who wanted to maintain their health, we would do an active practice. But, for those who were symptomatic and sick, we would do a gentle practice, and I would support them with pillows and blankets. I incorporated guided imagery, touch, energy work, meditation, and things I'd learned in Dr. Carl Simonton's work, which was so important in my own healing. Dr. Simonton was a radiation oncologist who popularized the mind-body connection in cancer and disease.

I combined all this, and became a certified yoga therapist as well. When I moved to Santa Barbara, I started therapeutic yoga and began teaching the program at Ridley Tree Cancer Center. I've been there 20 years, teaching weekly classes for the patients. My specialty is cancer, and I work privately, on Zoom with people all over the world. And now, I teach training in therapeutic yoga for those who want to become certified, and share healing through this beautiful practice that brought me back to myself.

Julia: How did you meet Laura Huxley?

Cheri: When I was sick I read one of her books and it had a huge impact on me. Laura Huxley, the widow of Aldous Huxley, was an amazing woman, a psychotherapist, and author.

I was in a grocery store, and I saw a woman who looked like the woman on the back of the book I was reading. I walked up to her and said, "Are you Laura Huxley?"

She said, "Yes" and I said, "You really helped me! I was terribly ill, and your book, This Timeless Moment, was a turning point." She took my hand, and we chatted and she invited me for tea. When I walked into her home about a week or so later, she said, "You need to scream," and I said, "What?"

She said, "You haven't found your voice, you need to scream," and I am a little startled, standing there in her foyer. So, I screamed, this small sound coming out of my throat. She said "No, do it again," and I let out this primal scream, to which she said, "Oh, that's good, now we can have tea."

That was the beginning of a beautiful 23-year relationship, where I ended up teaching her yoga and she wrote a lovely piece for my book. We became very close. I was with her when she was dying. She taught me so much about aging gracefully; she hiked in the hills and had a treadmill in front of her TV. She never just sat around, ever. She would stand on one foot as she talked on the phone, she did tai chi, and mediated, and was also clean with her diet—very thoughtful. If you had dinner, she would cut and serve only fruit for dessert, nothing else. She was vegetarian, an extraordinary, elegant soul. She taught me so much.

Julia: Now, you teach teachers to teach?

Cheri: With my co-teacher, Arturo Peal, we've been teaching for 23 years. We started in New York City where doctors and nurses said, "We need this in the hospitals!" That was always my goal, to take yoga to people who didn't think they could do yoga—to make it accessible to everyone. This practice is about meeting the needs of the person, rather than the person fitting into the practice.

I learned that early on, working with those with HIV and AIDS, that they needed the practice to be suited for them. Yoga is about listening and honoring the body, and being kind to one's self. It's not about pushing. The body speaks through sensation, and we must always listen, and if there's a "**No,**" we back off. The practice is a beautiful time of garnering and gaining a relationship with this amazing body. The Yogis say the body is the temple of the spirit, one that needs to be loved and cared for so that we can have grace. Both you and I know what it's like to be sick as kids, and struggle in pain, suffer, and for some *of us, helping others becomes our mission. We are the wound-ed healers. I see that in my training all the time. We have peo-ple who have been through extraordinary illness and healing, and they want to help others. We can help each other! We don't have all the answers, so we need each other's support.*

Julia: What do we say to people who see yoga as intimidat-ing? How do they find something suited to them, wherever they're at?

Cheri: *They can call a yoga center, and be honest, and say, "I have a back issue," and maybe they'll discover the center has a class specifically designed to heal the back. The studio might offer a restorative class. And, don't be afraid to do taste test-ing. Go to a few classes. If you're in a class and it's too much, don't worry, you don't have to do what the teacher is doing. You can lay down and rest, or go into child's pose; you don't have to keep up. I think now, more than ever, yoga teachers are aware that people have gone through trauma, or illness, and are healing, or haven't been to a class in a long time. Some yoga teachers are trained in trauma-informed yoga, and know how to be sensitive.*

Actually, that is what yoga is about. When yoga first came to America, it was taught differently. You would lie on your back and do shavasana, or rest, in between each pose, and just feel into what was happening. Now, the poses move along, they flow to some degree, and if it's moving too fast, it can be over-whelming. You don't have to keep up. Just enjoy where your body is, and if one class doesn't work for you, try another.

I do monthly workshops when I'm not doing teacher train-ings, and my husband plays live music and I teach a nourishing, stress reducing class. Everyone is welcome. My teacher train-ing sessions on Zoom now have people from all over the world, and I am so happy about that.

Julia: Thank you!

Cheri: I feel like women desperately need the information that you're sharing, because there needs to be a voice speaking through the quagmire of negative messaging about aging. I speak about that in my classes, that our scars and our wrinkles, they carry what we've lived through, and they are to be celebrated, not hidden. Of course, we want to feel our best. We want to look beautiful and love how we look.

Julia: Yes, and every woman has to decide what that means to her. We don't believe in judgment or shame. We do feel if every woman was healthy, happy, and strong, she would feel more self-acceptance, and have less of a need for invasive procedures. But, if an eye lift makes someone feel completely renewed, who are we to judge?

Cheri: Yes! That reminds me of a documentary I saw on plastic surgery. They featured a woman who was a crime scene photographer, and she said she felt all the pain she had ever witnessed on her face. After she had the surgery, she said, "Oh, that's who I am, that's me." There are so many reasons why people choose what they do, and it's important to honor every person's path.

Laura Huxley used to ask, "Why do we think self-care is selfish? Women are taught taking care of yourself is selfish, but it is the opposite. You're not only doing it for yourself, but for everyone around you. if you're healthy, you won't get sick and need care, and you can be self-sufficient longer." She would say, "Self-care is a gift you give to the people who love you," and that is so profound. We are supposed to mother and care for everyone, but we forget about ourselves. As for me, my co-teacher came to my office one day many years ago, and looked at my calendar. He said, "Where are your days off?"

I said, "I don't have any, too many people need help." He said, "If you don't take care of yourself, you're going to burn out," and he started making x's on my days. I started to feel what it was like to make space—it was a turning point for me. I have *a day off now, every week, and I take baths, with oils; I hike, go to the ocean, read, meditate, do yoga, and make good smoothies. I have to take the advice I give others.*

You can find Cheri at therapeuticyoga.com and her trainings at therapeuticyogatraining.com.

Pilates, Master of Precision, and Control

At the turn of the century, Joseph Pilates created an exquisite system for developing control, flexibility, balance, and alignment. Now, enjoyed by millions worldwide as a transformational exercise, Pilates stretches and strengthen muscles, and focuses on core strength.

The son of a naturopath and gymnast, Pilates was inspired to create strength building exercises while he was a prisoner of war (POW) during WWI on the Isle of Man. Practicing on fellow internees, the goal was to help them stay strong, even if emotionally or physically weakened. Some barely able to walk, he created exercises that could be done from a prone position—leg lifts, arm circles, and pelvic tilts.

After the war, Pilates designed equipment to support movement practices. *Reformer*, is his most well-known apparatus—a table-like bed attached to weights and pulleys. This apparatus allows anyone to build strength through resistance training. As strength builds, resistance is increased by adding heavier springs or weights. Based on the principles of *Classic Pilates*, a number of Pilates versions are taught today. There are generally two kinds of classes: Reformer and mat classes. Both focus on the practice of precise, controlled movements. These exercises stretch and strengthen muscles, protect bones, and improve posture. When taking a Reformer class, don't be intimidated by the look of the machine, with its straps and springs! This contraption will guide you to flex your body, as you use weights as resistance. If you want to build core strength, this is a phenomenal system.

In a mat class, you cultivate the same precise, slow movements to strengthen and stabilize your core, while also straightening the spine. The first aspect you will notice is the instructor's attention to detail. Precision is an essential facet of Pilates, one of the safest forms of exercise for anyone of any age. Many are drawn to Pilates to heal injuries caused by less detail oriented movement practices. The goal is for precision to become second nature and for the body to automatically move with grace and fluidity. One telltale sign of aging is the shift from sensual to stiff, robotic movements. To watch famed ballerina Margot Fonteyn as she dances Swan Lake in her late fifties—you would guess she was 35. When we reclaim flexibility and strength, we exhibit a youthful charisma.

Pilates is known for:

- Calming the nerves
- Relieving chronic pain
- Reducing inflammation
- Increasing metabolic rate
- Decreasing your waistline
- Creating lean muscle mass
- Improving range of motion
- Healing back and neck pain
- Building strength and flexibility
- Tightening your core and flattening your belly

Pilates taught me to move deliberately, which has resulted in shifts in how I move and think. For example, as a multitasker, I am always doing too many things at once. Therefore, I fall over the curb, and am prone to push *send* before proofreading an email or notice to whom the note is being sent. Slowing down has been a challenging, yet a worthy lesson. Pilates demands attention to detail—and the reward is a strong sense of dominion.

Control has become a less attractive word than it once was, less desirable than *surrender* or *acceptance*. However, to be in control of one's life, to be "the captain of our own ship," as Patricia Bragg would say, doesn't have to mean rigidity or denial. The more we take control of what we *can* control— such as our breath, food, and drink—the stronger and more flexible we are when the world tosses us into a storm from which we rebound, like the *Unsinkable Molly Brown*. These practices are the building blocks, the foundation, of a sea-worthy ship. We may have to batten down the hatches and occasionally change course, but we discover a new world in the process. We become more of who we were born to be.

Action Steps

1. Start with a gentle yoga class at home by streaming one of the online options at the back of this book. Just double up a blanket lengthwise, or buy an inexpensive mat to start. You can use home tools as aids, such as a firm pillow instead of a yoga bolster or even a stack of books instead of yoga blocks to help you reach the floor in forward bends, if necessary. As you start a regular practice, you may want to join a yoga studio that provides or rents yoga tools, or you may want to buy a starter set available online or in big box stores. And, as you strengthen and become more flexible, you may not even need the tools.

2. Try Pilates at home by starting with a streaming mat class, which requires no equipment. Pay close attention to the instructor's descriptions of how to hold a position and for how long. Use any home tools recommended or go to an introductory class at a Pilates studio in your area. Because Pilates is about using your muscles in precisely prescribed ways, it is often beneficial to work with an instructor in person to start to learn the minute details of a correct position in an exercise. Once you do, you will be surprised to find yourself remembering the correction when doing mat classes at home.

Revolutionary Beauty Barbara Gates

Meet Revolutionary Beauty Barbara Gates, a former Fortune 500 executive, who healed her body, mind, and spirit with the Bragg Healthy Lifestyle, lymphatic drainage therapy, colonics, and a life changing yoga practice.

Barbara: *I grew up studying my mother's beautiful fashion magazines—Vogue, Bazaar, Town & Country. I longed to grow up looking like these cool, long, and lanky, sophisticated women I saw.*

However, I learned early in life that I didn't live up to the female body portrayed in the pages of the magazines. All through grade school I was the tallest of all the kids in the class including the boys, and I was bigger, chunkier. As I got older, I looked nothing like the slender, angular bodies on the fashion runway. I had rounded curves (which I now embrace fully), not angles. And, by the way, I was never overweight. I was just big kid.

Although I never had an eating disorder, I definitely engaged in psychological self-harming. I imagined that every boy I liked who didn't like me, simply thought I was fat. I imagined that the popular girls would like me and I would be popular, too, if only I wasn't so big. I was a complete stranger to the self-love I have for myself now at 55 years old.

I also had a very angry, verbally abusive, domineering father. His constant message to me was that I was definitely not good enough. My vicious internal critic found a backup chorus of negativity in him, and I believed it. After moving out of the house to begin my own life, I began working in the film industry. You guessed it, I was faced with an even deeper level of self judgement and body image issues that I could not keep up with, even in a behind-the-cameras work of script or story development. I had a boyfriend I met at the Sundance Film Festival who I initially adored, but soon he started to speak to me as abusively as my father.

It was a turning point for me. I suddenly realized that I couldn't buy into how he saw me. True story. I moved out and away from him within days. But, it took years to end my negative, judgmental self-talk, and come to a place of self compassion and love. My turning point came in 2009, I endured a botched lumbar spine fusion surgery that left me in high pain, and in bed for years. During that time, the pain was much more intense than the pain that was to be remedied by the surgery itself. In 2012, I had a major spine fusion to correct it all. I began to believe that I could get out of bed, off all opiates, Ambien, and Klonopin, and get back to living a normal life. The seven-and-a-half-hour surgery was intense.

For my body, heart, mind, and spirit, it was devastating—like sustaining wounds on a battlefield. I couldn't sit up for more than about 15 minutes without pain. The pain had become chronic. I suffered from medical trauma post-traumatic stress disorder (PTSD), and had nightmares and disturbing daytime flash backs. I suffered from adrenal fatigue. I even bought a couple of walking canes thinking that I'm disabled. I began to get epidural shots every few months for pain and was hardly able to leave my bed. Then, another disc suddenly split, causing terrible additional pain.

My hopes of getting back to a normal life were destroyed. Fusion surgery number three was done in early 2014 to remove yet another "bad disc." I suddenly became determined to start doing yoga. It was a persistent thought and I felt driven to do it, even with a spine fused from my waist to my sacrum. I met an excellent yoga teacher who became a wellness coach for me. It took about four years of yoga, often practicing in pain, but continuing to keep trying until I started to declare that I was "out of chronic pain." It took years of dedication and continuing to show up on the mat. In addition to yoga, including breathing exercises and meditation, I radically changed how I ate—gluten-free, dairy-free, and mostly organic with lots of food-as-medicine vegan meals. I still eat chicken and fish, but I am having more and more plant based meals each week.

I have moved my body from an acidic internal environment to a much healthier alkaline one. I drink and cook with bone broth for gut health. I make sure I am eating lots of plant based foods each day and drink a ton of alkaline water. I have an infrared sauna, and I get lymphatic massages and colonics to remove waste and toxins that collect in the body from years of poor diet and medications.

I am happy, healthy, and completely healed!

Revolutionary Beauty Elaine LaLanne

The epitome of Revolutionary Beauty, Elaine LaLanne is still doing push-ups at 95. A dear friend of Patricia for decades, she met her late husband, Jack, when he appeared on a television show she hosted. Her husband, Jack LaLanne, was a sickly, suffering teenager when he met Paul Bragg at a lecture. Jack immediately devoted himself to the Bragg Healthy Lifestyle, which not only healed his body, but ignited his passion for fitness. Jack became a household name, and started gyms across America, inventing juicers, and getting America off the couch. He met his match with Elaine, one of the first ladies of television, an unstoppable powerhouse with a great sense of humor.

Elaine: *I'm headed for 95! I guess I'd be in the category of representing ageless fitness.*

When I met Jack, I was on a 90-minute television show. My position was called Girl Friday. *Today, I'd be called a cohost. I booked all the guests, and also appeared for 90 minutes live. When I was on the* Today Show *with my first book,* Fitness After 50, *there were three-minute segments, and they had one person interview me. When I first worked in TV, I did the whole show. It was in 1948, and that was when TV first started.*

When I first started in TV, it didn't come on till 6 pm. We later went on at 4:30 pm, and was called The Les Malloy Show.

In 1953, I left TV. Les Malloy, my boss, bought a radio station and I learned to do everything; I learned to run the whole station.

When I met Jack, I was 27. I would come in early at 9 am; I'd walk in with my donut and my bearclaw, and he came over and said, "You know you should be eating apples, bananas, and OJ, and if I didn't like you, I wouldn't tell you that."

I took a puff of my cigarette, blew smoke at him and said, "Oh yeah?"

He said to me, "The only thing good about the donut is the hole in the middle!"

Jack took 30 pounds off a guy in 30 days on his show—I was impressed—and he started an exercise class at noon, so I started exercising. I was in the Aqua Follies in the early 1940s so I was a ballet swimmer, and I grew up in Minneapolis, and you never think about exercising to take off weight or anything, you just eat. That's what we did in those days.

After I joined the class, one day he brought over a picture of pink and black lungs, and I said, "I'm 27, I don't want lungs with holes." Jack's brother came by and said, "It takes a year to get the nicotine out of your lungs." I quit! Right then, I quit. And, I changed the way I ate; I started broiling everything instead of frying, and eating healthier and healthier.

I had been married once before; I thought I was done with men. I didn't date Jack till 1953. We went together six years before we were married. I didn't rush. We got married in 1959.

He taught me everything I know today, and of course, Paul Bragg changed his life at 14. Paul and Patricia—we used to see them all the time. Paul was on Jack's show, and I met Patricia, and we'd go out to dinner. We've been close ever since.

I kept up that way of living. At 80, I have let myself have a bite of something fun here and there. When I turned 80, I said, "Jack, you know I've been good all this time; I haven't had anything but healthy food since we met. I'm 80 and if it's a birthday, I'm going to have a bite of cake!"

Jack said, "It's not what you do some of the time that counts; it's what you do most the time."

In my book, If You Want to Live, Move! Putting the Boom Back in the Boomers, *we have an 80-percent-rule. We want the boomers to get going again, as some have gone by the wayside. We have a plan to start out with eight minutes a day of exercise. Eight minutes a day gets you on your way.*

Now, Jack **never** *deviated. He would never eat anything that wasn't good for him. He said, "That's my feeling. I don't ask people to do as I do. I only ask them to try for most of the time;" he advocated for "most of the time."*

I'm writing a book, Try and Discipline; the Legacy of Jack La-Lanne in His Own Words and Those He's Inspired. *Of course, Paul Bragg is in there, and Arnold Schwarzenegger, and Patricia Bragg, and Keith Morrison from Dateline—he knew Jack—and many golfers and fans. Clint Eastwood was a Bragg fan. Patricia's brother went to school with him. Clint worked out with Jack.*

Julia: Elaine, you have gorgeous skin! What are your beauty secrets?

Elaine: *I took care of my skin, always. I always put moisturizer on it. I made my own. I don't make it anymore, but Jack created a cream, Moisture Tone, and we decided we'd come out with it, and that was in 1955. We've had it ever since. It's all natural.*

I don't fast now, but I did. I didn't do it as often as Paul and Patricia did, nor did I do water fasts. I did a watermelon fast with Jack. We ate so much watermelon. When we got hungry, we'd go to a movie and eat our watermelon. Jack loved fasting. He was a huge proponent of it. I also sleep well; not as long as I used to. I try to get eight, but it's usually seven. Sleep is important.

Julia: Elaine, what are your goals?

Elaine: *To get this book done and have Jack LaLanne get his due; and a documentary as well. That's my goal, and then, I'm ready to go. You have three ages—chronological age, physical age (how you feel), and psychological age. Forget the chronological and concentrate on the other two.*

Julia: What is your psychological age?

Elaine: *It used to be 19 and now it's 39! Jack Benny's age.*

Julia: What is your physical age?

Elaine: *My physical age would be 39, too.*

Julia: What is a tip about how to feel your best?

Elaine: *When people are turning 40, 50, 60, some think that's over the hill. You're just beginning. Make a checklist. Write down all your negative thoughts about your age; and about your life. Then, make another list, and then, write all the positive things. Do you want to be positive or negative?*

If you're depressed, think how much you learned on the earth. At times you worry and worry, and a year later you can't even remember what you worried about. Do the check list.

I believe in introspection. Look inside every day. Don't get stuck in the past. Yesterday is gone and tomorrow isn't here yet.

Jack said, "Right now is the most important time of your life. You can't live in the last minute or the next minute."

*It's very important. Don't let criticism bother you. **You** know who you are. It's just going to make you miserable. And, don't make excuses. This happened, "I'm sorry"—tell the truth. The only thing constant is change. Don't worry about making excuses.*

*I've lived a long time and learned a lot. We all learn from some-body else. I learned from Jack; he learned from me; he learned from Paul; if we interact together, we learn from each other. And, we continue to learn till we die. There's **so much** to learn in life!*

MODULE 6

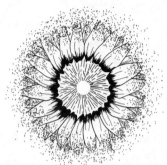

Episode 12
HORMONES & SENSUALITY

"Hormones shape who we are."

—Suzanne Somers, Trailblazing Health Educator
and Best-Selling Author

Hormone balance is essential to ageless beauty. Stress and environmental toxins play havoc with hormone health. This leads to gut issues, weight gain, fatigue, and depression. Dr. Michael Galitzer, MD, says, "From the perspective of medicine, the word "hormone" means to *arouse and excite*." Who feels sexy while they struggle with brain fog and burnout?

Bioidentical hormones and herbal remedies were not available for our grandmothers. Nevertheless, they generally didn't need them, either. While most of us would not trade the freedom to be fully ourselves for our grandmother's social limitations, present-day hormones are deeply affected by environmental toxicity. Painful periods, endometriosis, and polycystic ovary syndrome (POS) affect an entire generation of young women. One of three couples in America between 25 and 45 struggle with infertility. More often than not, perimenopausal and menopausal women describe *the change of life* as "a nightmare." You do not need to suffer. Safe and effective solutions are available for these challenges. In truth, this is the best time in history to be a woman. When I began my career, my menopausal clients had two main options to reduce their mood swings, hot flashes, and fatigue. One was Premarin, a toxic hormonal medication made from horse urine that caused cancer. The other choice was the *grin-and-bare-it approach*. For some, herbal formulas worked well—but not for all.

As I witnessed the dawn of hormone replacement therapy (HRT), through my client's grateful stories, I knew a new day was upon us. Suzanne Somer's revolutionary books opened the information floodgates. I met pioneering doctors who formulated safe and effective herbal remedies for women. When a prospective client called in agony over mood swings and weight gain, I knew I could offer solutions.

Most importantly, I want you to know that many options are available to you now. Many clients experience life changing results with natural, bioidentical hormone supplements. Others find relief through herbal, homeopathic, and naturopathic formulas. We do not advocate any one modality. Each woman's body is different. Genetics, lifestyle, and health history are critical to choosing which hormonal support system may work.

If you experience any of the symptoms listed, please contact a doctor or practitioner. Do not endure another day. If one doctor's technique and presentation does not feel right, get a second or third opinion. Be patient with the process. To balance hormones is a dance that takes time. Hormone protocols are not a simple, one-size-fits-all prescription. Finding an expert whom you trust is imperative.

Perimenopausal and Menopausal Symptoms

Do you find any of your symptoms in the following list?

Low Estrogen

- Spotting
- Insomnia
- Bone loss
- Headaches
- Hot flashes
- Depression
- Low energy
- Decreased libido
- Irregular periods
- Fatigue
- No "glow"
- Weight gain
- Mood swings
- More wrinkles
- Vaginal dryness
- Painful intercourse
- Risk of heart disease
- Urinary tract infections

Low Progesterone

- Anxiety
- Fibroids
- Migraines
- Headaches
- Depression
- Endometriosis
- Low libido
- Hot flashes
- Weight gain
- Mood changes
- Irregular periods
- Thyroid dysfunction

Low Testosterone

- Anxiety
- Depression
- Weight gain
- Mood swings
- Dry or thinning skin
- Decreased sex drive
- Loss of muscle mass
- Difficulty climaxing
- Reduced bone density
- Difficulty losing weight
- Exhaustion and fatigue
- Difficulty concentrating
- Short-term memory loss

Low Thyroid

- Fatigue
- Dry skin
- Hoarseness
- Constipation
- Puffy face
- Weight gain
- Sensitivity to cold
- Muscle weakness

If you know or suspect that you are exhibiting thyroid issues contact a doctor or specialist. Do not try to treat yourself. Blood tests can provide definitive answers.

Shifting Hormones

Hormones dictate levels of aliveness and vibrancy. Though hormone levels shift throughout life, we are more directly impacted after 50. We can grit our teeth through menopause, or glide. My choice to be proactive is one of the best decisions I ever made. Balancing hormones safeguards bones, protects memory, mental clarity, and boosts energy. If you are frustrated by weight gain, hormone support may shift this in a way that exercise alone does not. Patience, creativity, and joy depend on endocrine system strength—as does Vital Force. We are only as happy and healthy as our hormones are balanced.

Adrenal Support

The thyroid and adrenal glands are also affected by menopause. If you are exhausted all the time, no matter what you do, that is adrenal fatigue. Adrenal fatigue is epidemic in America—85 percent of my female clients exhibit symptoms of this debilitating condition. No surprise, as stress is the number one enemy to adrenals—followed by diet and lifestyle choices.

Symptoms of Adrenal Fatigue

- Brain fog
- Gut issues
- Inability to sleep
- Small things upset you
- Dark circles under eyes
- Catch colds and flues easily
- Dizzy when you stand up
- Decreased (or no) sex drive

- Feelings of fear and sadness
- Constant state of exhaustion

Sleep does not refresh or energize. These beautiful warriors are tired, frustrated, and confused. Some feel utter despair. To that end, well-meaning doctors or therapists prescribe antidepressants. While this may be helpful short-term, if adrenal fatigue is the source, medication will not fix the problem. I interviewed esteemed endocrine specialists for their strategy to heal adrenal fatigue.

They recommended the following:

1. Stress reduction
2. Detoxification
3. Nutritional support
4. Exercise
5. Hormone balance and adrenal support

In other words, this is the "The CARE Plan," which meets the requirements to create optimal health. These savvy doctors understand that detoxification must precede supplementation for optimal results. Otherwise, organs are so overwhelmed that even correctly prescribed supplements increase symptoms, rather than alleviate them.

If your hormones are circling the drain, diet alone may not be enough to boost your adrenals. Vitamins, minerals, enzymes, and adrenal treatment speeds recovery. Natural sleep formulas aid rest and recuperation.

To heal adrenal fatigue, follow this list of suggestions:

- Stay hydrated
- Reduce alcohol
- Minimize caffeine
- Prioritize stress reduction
- Allow yourself to rest when tired

- Carve solo time into your calendar
- Take food enzymes with each meal
- Sleep seven hours a night, minimum
- Meditate and practice deep breathing
- Drink protein shakes in between meals
- Avoid sugar and high fat processed foods
- Consume 50-100 grams of digestible protein daily

Start with Detoxification

Revolutionary Beauty's mindfulness, purification, and dietary practices dramatically reduce inflammation and allow the endocrine system to heal. The doctors with whom I work recommend we implement these, which allows for less yet more effective supplementation. Everything we ingest that is not food or juice is strenuous for the body to assimilate—particularly the liver. Hormone supplementation is frequently prescribed in cream form—since the skin is the largest organ, and easily absorbs these formulas.

Hormone balance is highly relevant to ageless beauty, no matter your age. We are vulnerable to hormone issues throughout life—whether menopause is a distant memory, or if you are still menstruating. Women are goddesses of adaptation. Yet, immeasurable stress and toxicity have taxed our ability to thrive in this modern world. Save your grit for the battles that call for endurance, strength, and tenacity. Menopausal symptoms need not be one of them. Whether through herbal formulas, homeopathic, or bioidentical HRT, expect to feel like a new person within weeks. Do not become accustomed to doing your best with whatever hormones remain. A slight tweak of these levels has the power to change your life in ways you cannot imagine.

Action Steps

1. Keep a journal of your *symptoms* of menopause or perimenopause, including date, time, and length

(i.e. of hot flashes). Review with your gynecologist or naturopath (or both) and discuss treatment options.
2. Read about the pros and cons of each option to make an informed decision.
3. Try which option you feel is best. If you don't get the results you want, don't be afraid to try another.

In Conclusion

Balancing your hormones, including thyroid and adrenals, may be the shift you are looking for to boost your:

- Mood
- Libido
- Energy
- Optimism
- Muscle tone
- Bone density
- Skin elasticity
- Collagen levels

And reduce your:

- Inflammation
- Thin skin and wrinkles
- Brain fog and memory loss
- Feelings of fear and anxiety

Revolutionary Beauty Dr. Leigh Connealy, MD

Practicing since 1986, Dr. Leigh Connealy, MD is a prominent leader in the field of Integrative Medicine, the founder and director of the Center for New Medicine and the Cancer Center for Healing in Irvine, California. The two clinics combined have become the largest integrative medical clinics in North America and have been visited by over 47,000 patients.

Dr. Connealy uses the best of sciences, including conventional, western medicine, homeopathic, eastern medicine, and the new modern medicine. She is the author of two books we highly recommend, *The Cancer Revolution*, and *Be Perfectly Healthy*, (also the brand name of her health and skincare products) that have revolutionized the landscape of medicine. In 2017 and 2021, she was named one of the top 50 functional and integrative medical doctors in America. Dr. Connealy's compassion and understanding comes not only from treating thousands of patients, but her own health history as a diethylstilbestrol (DES) baby. The DES drug taken by her mother created health challenges for her like hormonal problems, fertility challenges, and anatomical issues.

In 2019, Dr. Connealy endured a total of 18 hours of back surgeries in Germany to correct a congenital condition, lifelong scoliosis in her back which also stemmed from being a DES baby. She says she will never retire, as her desire is to help as many people heal as possible. Cancer, now an epidemic worldwide, affects one of three women and one of two men. She is happily married, a grandmother, and the mother of a combined family of seven children. She tells her friends and patients, "Happiness and true satisfaction comes from experiencing every facet of life."

Dr. Connealy: *I'm not just a doctor who went to school to research and study. I have done that, but I have also had health challenges and life interruptions that have opened my eyes and made me question everything. I know there are people out there who have had a great normal life, who have never been sick or struggled. I think that is great, but that has just not been my experience; I don't wish ill health on anyone, but you are only awakened in the valley.*

Julia: How did you heal from your 18 hours of back surgeries?

Dr. Connealy: *First, there is the preparation. I prepared for three months in advance. I focused on the mental aspect* with visualization and affirmations—how this was going to go, how whole and healthy I would be after. Then, I did hyperbaric, weekly vitamin IVs, saunas, nutritional prescriptions, and self-healing. I prep every patient for every surgery, no matter what it is, with nutrient supplementation, hyperbaric treatments, IV protocols, and we focus on their psycho-mental-emotional well-being. Personally, I said a Novena prayer before surgery and afterwards. For me, spirituality is key to everything, and especially to healing.

Mentally we have to program ourselves. I have gotten good at that now. I learned about that only ten years ago. I have studied all facets of mental and emotional well-being and have brought different aspects of that into my life and into my work. After my surgery, as soon as I got home, I immediately started hyperbaric treatments, immunity boosting IVs, maintained a perfect nutrition plan, did lots of daily green drinks, and added supplementation. Then, I had to do an anti-candida protocol because the antibiotics all gave me candida. Because my gut was a mess from the antibiotics and the meds, I got parasites and needed to focus on that as well, so I did all kinds of bioenergetic restoration. I am doing amazingly well now. I am working out every day, lifting weights, walking, stretching. From where I came from, this is truly a miracle!

I tried everything for years to reverse my scoliosis condition before I chose surgery. I know a lot about pain and the reversal of structure now. I would not have learned that if I just took a course because living it is quite different. You learn it—you live it. The experience teaches you tremendous discipline and compassion for humanity, and you have no choice but to be positive; being negative doesn't get you anywhere. Being negative changes your vibration, literally. I am a perennial student, and even though my back is fixed; I read constantly about healing and pain management. I am always learning.

I have tried to eliminate stress, strife, and struggle, and all kinds of innovative strategies which are crucial to healing and being healthy. I have been through a lot, and I am on a mission to educate and empower people to truly work on their health. Your health needs to be your number one value.

Julia: What are your tips for longevity and ageless beauty?

Dr. Connealy: *Live in gratitude and believe that nothing is impossible. Don't be overwhelmed because life is overwhelming. There is always going to be something in front of you to deal with. But focus on joy—happiness makes you beautiful. I'm not saying every moment every day you're going to be happy, because you're not. Every day say, "I can accomplish whatever I want, whatever I need to do," because that changes not only you, but your body—physically, mentally, emotionally, energetically. Words that you say to yourself are powerful. Turn every negative into a positive. I started this a long time ago, and when I did, my life changed. Say, "I want to be different. I am going to make a conscious effort to be different." And maybe, if you didn't have difficult situations, you would not have learned that lesson. Happiness comes from within—how you live your life every day.*

Julia: What habits do you teach that promote health and happiness?

Dr. Connealy: *Sleep affects your mood. We must sleep. Drink water. Eat foods that make you healthy. If you eat lots of desserts and dead food; your body can't be alive; every cell is alive taking care of you 24/7. Take supplements daily to maintain your health. We live in an outrageously toxic world, being sick is very expensive, especially emotionally.*

If you don't schedule your health, your illness will schedule you. I have a front row seat to disaster every single day—people in the worst situations possible. Many of my patients are diagnosed with stage-four cancer. How did they get there?

There are things that you have to do that may seem crazy, like coffee enemas, but those have been around a long, long time, and they are part of detoxification, so critical to health in a toxic world. Hippocrates said, "it all starts in the colon." A doctor in Portugal, Dr. Serge Jurasunas, wrote an incredible book called Health and Disease Begins in the Colon.

Sixty percent of the population is chronically ill. We need to all be up in arms about that. Until we decide health is number one from the beginning, from birth, we can't be a healthy world, a healthy nation, a healthy family. Health is everything.

Julia: Patricia Bragg says, "Your health is your wealth." And she talks about love and kindness as components of health.

Dr. Connealy: *Love is the medicine for everything, so we have to be gentle when we speak and teach—not be too domineering and forceful. We must talk about what works for us. Compassion must lead. Nothing else heals if people don't feel loved.*

Julia: Do you offer aesthetics at your clinic?

Dr. Connealy: *Absolutely, we do all kinds of things. And, I use everything I create on myself first, of course. Recently, I received a facial treatment whereby I spun my blood to isolate the growth factors and mixed it with exosomes and placenta stem cells and injected it in my face. It is fantastic. I am against plastic surgery unless you have a congenital deformity. Beauty is an inside job. People want a quick fix, and they get consumed with trying to look like they are 25 years old. Enjoy being who you are. You can do a lot of noninvasive enhancements before surgery. I'm coming out with a line of skin products that is being formulated in Italy using plant exosomes to repair your skin and your body. I hope to roll out in 2022. I will have a body cream with exosomes; that is what I am working on now.*

I know many women who have breast implants want them out after 50, and some even younger, for health issues. We know it's a foreign object that our bodies must contend with. Watch the documentary, bOObs. *Just be aware and investigate before adding a foreign body into your system. Another tip: there are different opinions and studies on underwire bras and the safety of them; but I explain to my patients that studies have also shown that the wire may constrict your lymph glands and may cause inflammation. It is just something to keep in mind when selecting a bra.*

Julia: Patricia Bragg has been preaching that for 50 years. What are your thoughts on hormone replacement therapy?

Dr. Connealy: *I believe that all people need hormones, men and women. Especially after menopause and andropause, all men and women need bioidentical hormone replacement. Correctly formulated, it's safe. At an oncology meeting that I attended, doctors presented documentation that estrogen does not cause breast cancer. Every one of us needs bioidentical hormones; they are essential molecules that our body needs, especially because of the environment. I have lived the hormonal conundrum myself, so I know what it's about to wonder what should be done, which led to the intense amounts of study I have done on the subject. And, when I say we all need hormones, I do not just mean female hormones, but **all** of them—adrenal, pituitary, testosterone, estrogen, thyroid, everything. Every one of them is important. They all need support. But, hormonal issues don't just affect women over 50. You may have hormonal problems at any age; even 25-years-old, because there are so many endocrine disruptors changing how our whole body works. Rachel Carlson wrote the book, Silent Spring, and everything she said is happening!*

Julia: Did you know that Paul Bragg was an environmental advocate almost 100 years ago, and encouraged Rachel Carlson to write that book?

Dr. Connealy: *I didn't know that. I love that book. She was the beginning of bringing this information to mainstream America, and we are still trying to wake people up.*

MODULE 6

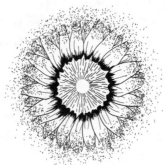

Episode 13
PLEASURE & ESSENCE

*"An inordinate passion for pleasure is
the secret to remaining young."*

—Oscar Wilde, Poet and Playwright

As we age, our relationship to sensuality and pleasure is richer, deeper, and more complex. Lovemaking is not the only path to pleasure. We seek a radical, joyful aliveness, and a wild passion for life, which we describe as *essence*. We see this essence in healthy teenagers. Sometimes to our chagrin, they fill the house with music, giggles, and nonstop lust for new, and often risky adventures. They live in the moment, capable of complete surrender to whatever brings pleasure.

In his wonderful book, *Brainstorm*, Dr. Daniel J. Siegel, MD, writes that the brain changes in adolescence as we incorporate four major qualities—which spell the word "essence."

- ES—Emotional Spark. Emotional intensity is a good description.
- SE—Social Engagement. Meaningful connections with others.

- N—Novelty. New experiences that fully engage us.
- CE—Creative Explorations. Expanded consciousness that creates a gateway to see the world through a new lens.

Dr. Siegel sees all of the above as critical for teens, as well as for adult health and happiness. He suggests that one reason adults conflict with teenagers is that grown-ups are disconnected from these essence rich qualities.

What is a room of teenagers compared to a room of adults? One is usually raucous and wild, bursting with booming music, loud laughs, and nonstop ideas. The other is predictably sedate. We all need balance. Yet, as we focused on career and family life, did we banish our *inner teen?*

The mind and body expects a carrot, a delicious reason to do the healing work. We need a reward, the way we might offer to take our children or grandchildren miniature golfing once their chores are completed. We can force ourselves to do almost anything for short periods of time. Humans were designed to be sprinters. However, we cannot run a marathon each day, day after day—we eventually break.

The soul-deep exhaustion many carry—and sadly labeled *failure* or *weakness*—eventually erodes desire. Both sensuality and sexuality is uniquely affected by this exhaustion. One of the reasons that 60-75 percent of my over 50 clients report sexual disinterest—even pleasuring themselves—is that they are tired *down to the bone*, physically, and emotionally. These mighty women have put their heads down and barreled ahead for so long, driven by obligation, and responsibility, that pleasure has become a foreign concept.

While a commitment to obligation is admirable, as a way of life, it is deadly. We modeled ourselves on the obsessive dynamics of our parents and culture—which developed unhealthy behaviors and relationship patterns in us:

- Codependent, unhealthy enmeshment with a loved one without autonomy
- Supporting or enabling a loved one's unhealthy behaviors
- Addiction to food, drugs, alcohol, shopping, or any self-sabotaging repetitive behavior
- Anger, resentment, and bitterness
- Depression and anxiety
- Martyrdom or over-responsibility for those seemingly unwilling or unable to care for themselves
- Denial and inability to see clearly what is happening
- Fight or flight—either fleeing a challenging situation or becoming too frozen to act
- Disassociation by not being present in our bodies
- Inability to take action on our own behalf or sustain self-care

Does any of this resonate with you?

You will notice this list matches many of the symptoms of brain injury discussed in "Module 1." A limbic system injury is often the reason we cannot identify these patterns when we're in the middle of them. Unconscious, they stem from a place of wounding—far from present time.

Of course, we struggle to *live in the moment*. When triggered, our mind flashes back to 1975 or 1995—a scene wherein we are paralyzed by the fear of retribution from an abusive partner or parent. Maybe we are seven-years-old, and dad just walked out the door. Or, we are 12, and the priest just told us that we're full of sin, or someone touched us inappropriately, and we are paralyzed. The hurts we have absorbed, trigger the past. No wonder we struggle to embody power as captivating a woman, in control of her beauty and sexuality.

Teenagers are ebullient because they getting a hefty dose of happiness hormones, thanks to Mother Nature. And, hopefully, they do not yet carry the weight of the world on their backs. (To the ones who are, we are sorry.) Most teenagers have not seen what you have seen. They have not fought the battles of juggling career and family life while balancing a budget, and navigating job loss, or divorce. When teens are healthy and loved, they are naturally bursting with joy and energy. This book is dedicated to the reclamation of that juicy nectar in you. Yet, juice runs low in a battery which needs to be recharged.

Mother Nature needs us to heal this planet. Our partners may long to make love, and enjoy time together. Yet, we cannot pour from an empty cup.

Do you remember how you felt about your face and body when you were a young adult? Most of us were so insecure and self-critical. Our breasts were too big or small, our hips too wide, and our faces pimpled and ravaged by the hormonal excesses we now miss. Few of us looked like *Cover Girl* models. Even Revolutionary Beauty Kelly LeBrock, says "I always thought I was too fat. And I hated my lips!" Can you imagine those were the fears of someone known as *the world's most beautiful woman?*

When you gaze at a picture of your younger self, I bet most of you are struck by how lovely you were. Sure, maybe your hairstyle seems humorous now. Regardless, looking into the eyes of that woman, you see her heart, soul, and potential. Maybe she is holding a world of hurt, and yet, has bolted into the fire anyway. How brave! She's lived, loved, and survived.

This woman deserves to feel pleasure, sensual, and sexual. If that statement takes you by surprise, I wish we could offer you a monthlong stay at an exquisite health spa. Mother Nature renews her warriors, and you are one of them. That is why "The CARE Plan" was created. As you breathe, meditate, purify, and move your body, your essence will rise. Your inner teen will reappear. She may not be the rebellious hellion she was, or the *good girl*, or the *silent girl*. Your inner teen will be fully integrated into the power of your present self. That is where pleasure begins.

You may be inspired to scribble notes about how to utilize your newfound energy. To your surprise, you will advocate, on your behalf, for exactly what you want. Without hesitation, you ask for support or advice. Finally, you discern to employ only what suits your unique path. If unclear, you wait. Time is on your side. When asked for help, you offer it only to those fighting for their life with the same commitment you have fought for yours. Everybody else is on their own. Feel the freedom!

To preserve your precious time and energy in this manner rebuilds Vital Force—the essence which is the foundation of desire. You will be amazed to feel delight stir as this process unfolds. *How* you enjoy that is up to you.

The Secret to Pleasure—Learning to Receive

If you graduated with honors from the *University of IBGTR*— "It's-better-to-give-than-receive"—it's time to shred that diploma! The perception that giving is, number one, always noble, and number two, always constructive, is false. In fact, giving—whether advice, money, or time—may do more harm than good.

When someone asks you for a favor, how quickly do you say "yes?" Do you ever allow yourself to hesitate, and examine the consequences and benefits?

The expectation that we should always give when asked— and give more than we receive—is a disaster for women. Due to these unhealthy expectations, many of us earned a PhD from the University of IBGTR by the time we were ten. As a result, we may not even know *how* to receive—let alone how our life might change if we learned.

202 Revolutionary Beauty by Julia Loggins with Patricia Bragg

"Put Down the Oars" is a visualization designed to teach receptivity and balance. When I first practiced this exercise, I realized the reason that I was often disappointed in past relationships—relationships of all kinds, not just romantic. While I longed for ease, I did not know that the secret to attainment came from doing less, not more.

In the visualization below, the partner in the boat with you may be anyone with whom you are close. Read the following aloud. Remember to breathe as you recite the words.

Put Down the Oars

Imagine you and your partner are sitting in a rowboat. You are both rowing the boat in the middle of a lake, on a warm summer afternoon. A basket of fresh fruit is tucked under your seat. As you have been rowing for a while, your arms have begun to ache. Put the oars down. Lean back. Resist the temptation to pick up the oars.

Observe. Does your partner automatically pick up the oars? If they don't, do you notice a tendency to want to grab them, for fear the boat may capsize, or go off-course? If so, don't touch the oars. Lean back. Do not fix this.

Take a bite from the fruit that is tucked under the seat. Shift your attention from your partner and enjoy the sun on your face. Notice if doing nothing makes you uncomfortable. Are you breathing deeply, or starting to pant? Is your mind racing? Are you putting a plan into place to row this boat back to shore? Do nothing. If you feel nervous, shake your hands and wrists. Shrug your shoulders up and down. Do not judge yourself. You cannot fail in this. This visualization is not a test of your character.

Choices are numerous. If your partner doesn't pick up the oars, do something other than fervently row. Initiate a conversation. Toss a seat cushion in their direction. Make a joke.

Humor is undervalued as a way to release tension and start a real conversation. The key is, choices exist.

Rowing solo is an exhausting way to live. I share that from firsthand experience. I do not blame my former partners. I was so fearful of rejection that I resisted putting the oars down long enough to give my partner a chance to pick them up—or not. I was not brave enough to let them fail, and sit with that uncertainty. When I began putting the oars down, my relationships transformed. And some ended.

For women and the world around them to be healthy, we must cultivate receptivity. The role of the masculine is to protect what the feminine creates. Mother Nature is the source of life, as are we.

While we spill tears over the loss of a coral reef, we may think of that faraway reef as a separate entity. Yet, no difference is discernible between that reef and ourselves. Mother Nature, our inner feminine, calls us to prioritize time and energy so that we may rebuild Vital Force. Doing so may feel wildly counterintuitive. Do it anyway. You will be rewarded with joy, creativity, imagination, pleasure, and ageless beauty.

Red Carpet Moments

Finding myself on red carpets was an odd experience for a flower child who colored her hair with five-dollar henna. Yet it gave me the opportunity to reexamine my self-worth. As Kenny and I departed the rented limo at my first ever Grammy Awards, I caught a glimpse of my face in the mirror. My cheeks were red and I resembled a boiled lobster. My palms were sweaty and I was barely breathing.

Focused on glamorous stars, the paparazzi were clamoring for a picture. One gentleman with a huge lens tapped me on my shoulder and said, "Hey, this night is about you, too. Look right here!" Startled, I thought, *maybe he's right.*

Through this photographer, Spirit spoke. I gathered my courage, took a breath, and smiled. My inability to feel worthy to receive, was not going to rob me of this moment.

I have reminisced over this scene many times, when my *small self* shrinks while offered a compliment or new opportunity. If I unconsciously resist the gifts in front of me, I ask myself, what message am I sending to the Universe?

My father, the son of Jewish Romanian refugees, worked seven days a week to forge a life of which he could be proud. On holidays, he adored giving my mom special presents, a necklace or winter coat. Each time she opened the gift, she smiled awkwardly, and stuffed the treasure back into the box. My father winced in disappointment and confusion. As a child, I saw my mother as ungrateful. As an adult, I realized she simply did not feel worthy.

If the Universe rolls out a red carpet, you belong there. Each of us is presented with red carpet moments. Sometimes we do not recognize them or see them for what they are. These moments may be disguised as too-good-to-be-true possibilities, people, or experiences. Trust that when you keep your pledge to prioritize yourself, unexpected gifts come your way. To receive them, lean back, and put down those oars.

As we prioritize self-care and open to the feminine, the more available we become to red carpet moments, and the doors they open. As you sashay down that aisle, *do it your way*. I did not carry a purse on Grammy Night. My glamorous accessory was a huge red cooler, packed with snacks, food, and juice. Those events are six hours long!

Your Discernment Meter

"Boundaries are the distance at which I can love you and me simultaneously."

—Prentis Hemphill

The ability to experience pleasure is tied to our ability to release inhibitions. Discernment helps us to build a foundation and erect boundaries which guarantee emotional safety. Though discernment should be a natural instinct, our discernment meter may be disconnected due to a limbic system injury. Your boundaries were violated and trust betrayed— including trust in yourself. As we heal our bodies, we need to recalibrate that discernment meter. We accomplish this through meditation, prayer, journaling, and time in nature. And, we learn to ask ourselves the right questions.

Become a 10!

On a scale of one to ten, how discerning are you? *One* denotes a woman who never says "no." She rises at dawn to work in a school cafeteria before her restaurant shift starts.

Immediately saying "yes" before weighing value versus cost is the flip side of never saying "no." The wrong "yes" and the wrong "no" are equally depleting.

The number *ten* signifies a Revolutionary Beauty who asks, "What is truly needed here?" or "Is this mine to do? Where is my time and energy best spent?" A *ten* might ask, "Is there actually anything that needs to be done?"

The number ten is often used to describe a physically perfect woman. Who can forget Bo Derek in the movie, *10*? Maybe we should repurpose the number 10 to describe a woman capable of true discernment. As we practice this art, years of stress melt from our face and body. Our skin glows! Having been *a one* most of my life, wisdom comes with age. The art of discernment is a lifetime journey, yet a worthy one. The ability to experience joy and pleasure depend on it.

If your discernment meter is rusty, don't hesitate to ask a trusted friend. Decisions need not be made in a vacuum. You are not alone. Ultimately, the final choice is always yours.

Reigniting Passion

"One thing I know to be true is when pleasure starts courting you, you have to eat it with your whole heart. Make space for it like a wild thing bursting into flames inside you. Throw yourself under the bus with joy. You have to gobble it completely whole. Don't wait for it to get better to enjoy it. If it finds its way to you in this rocky, sometimes downright horrific path, you've got to run straight toward it. Say, 'Hi, this is me, broken, beautiful, alive, in love, wrecked, and willing to dance with you again.'"

—Mariah Norris-Hale, *The Sky Inside*

Research shows, a woman's sexual peak occurs in the for-ties. Yet, women over 50 commonly feel a distinct lack of desire—even if in a loving relationship. Why? The common themes will not surprise you:

- Dryness
- Exhaustion
- Overwhelming stress
- Anxiety and depression
- Hormonal mood swings

Financial, health, career, and family related crises can create such immense stress that desire unexpectedly diminishes. When the crisis ends, desire isn't necessarily replenished. The yearning for intimacy is not controlled by a button or switch.

We can rediscover the power and delight of sensuality and sexuality. Sexuality and power are connected. Like sensuali-ty, sexuality does not equate only to the act of making love. Your sexuality is about feeling alive and passionate, and sat-isfied with your body. The *joie de vivre* energy that we re-member from youth is the gold at the end of the rainbow.

My client Jennifer, an architect, married with two sons, says, "Sex? It's been so long that I'm not sure I'd remember how to do it!" She laughs nervously, "It's not that I don't love Joe, I do. And it's not all me. There have been times when I was in the mood, and he wasn't. I guess that's frustrating, too. It's all confusing. It used to be so easy."

Truer words were never spoken. After 50, diminished hormones no longer put the *pedal to the metal*. We must consciously focus energy and attention toward this facet of life—or desire disappears.

Mary has been single for a decade. Though she loves her job at the nursery and describes herself as "overly self-sufficient," she misses being held. She is not sure she wants to remarry, or even live with anyone again. Regardless, Mary longs to find that special companionship in her life.

"We don't even need to have sex! Well, maybe I'm saying that because I've always been insecure about my desirability. My first husband left me for his partner's wife. If that doesn't hit you where you live, nothing does. But, I do remember a time, early in our marriage, when he couldn't wait to come home and get me into bed. It felt wonderful. Is it too late for that? Is that too much to hope for?"

I hear the yearning in her voice. She is not merely yearning for a partner. Mary is missing the experience of feeling fully alive. When she reclaims her sensuality, *Mr. or Ms. Right* will appear. That is how the Universe works—though not without a little footwork of our own. I met my wonderful husband through online dating. Though two close friends knew us both, neither had thought to introduce us.

Trust the process. Trust Mother Nature's timing. Be gentle with yourself. Let the metamorphosis continue. Autonomy, vitality, and creativity are key components of sexual and sensual aliveness. "The CARE Plan" fuels them all.

Prioritize Pleasure

Do you schedule time for pleasurable activities?

- Facials
- Massage
- Lovemaking
- Self pleasure
- Luxurious baths

We don't think twice about scheduling time for essentials like the dentist or accountant—maybe even *date night*. But, is date night a dinner out, or staying home and making love? Teenagers may be wired for sex at midnight, but the rest of us are not. In a research study, hundreds of couples were assigned the task of making love daily for 30 days. Nearly every couple reported a dramatic increase in each person's feelings of love and connection. Obviously, not all of these sessions included dinner and candlelight. Some were *quickies in the hallway.* Yet, when we don't feel sexually connected to our partner, a *quickie* may feel unsatisfying, rather than hot and exciting. *Use it or lose it* applies to sexuality as well as fitness!

The same is true with self pleasure. If we do not acknowledge what pleases us, it's only by sheer luck that a partner will hit gold. No one can read your mind. There are hundreds of self pleasuring toys on the market. If you haven't explored self pleasuring in a long time, you owe yourself the time and freedom to learn or relearn your own body. The body changes with every season. How you want to share your body is your choice.

Pleasure originates from the ability to receive. Abundance, opportunity, adventures, love, creativity, joy—these are all forms of pleasure. The endocrine system—as well as the gut and brain—is nourished by healthy, pleasurable sensations, and experiences. When we believe that positive thoughts heal, pleasure is the connector between neurotransmitters that reboot immunity. Pleasure is not frivolous. We do not need permission to cultivate pleasure. However, if you do, your wish is now granted!

Many excellent books written in the last decade on adult sexuality. Here are some I highly recommend:

- *Mating in Captivity* by Esther Perels
- *Vagina* by Naomi Wolf—author of *The Beauty Myth*
- *Conscious Loving Ever After, How to Create Thriving Relationships in the Second Half of Life* by Gay Hendricks, PhD and Kathlyn Hendricks, PhD

Pelvic Floor Therapy

Pelvic floor therapy liberated me from a lifetime of chronic bladder infections. This modality, a specialty of licensed physical therapists, frees the muscles in the pelvic region. These muscles can become either too relaxed or too tense, depending on the issue. Pelvic floor therapy is not painful, embarrassing, or invasive. I wish every woman could visit a pelvic floor therapist after childbirth, pelvic surgery, STDs, or sexual trauma—especially during menopause.

If you have never experienced an orgasm, a pelvic floor therapist may help more than your counselor or talk therapist. Possibly, the muscles inside your body may be too constricted to allow pleasure. Numerous clients of mine who never felt pleasure during sex, gained the ability to orgasm after pelvic floor therapy. Your body is not broken. You may only need the right kind of help and support. This is also true if you were once able to orgasm, but for some reason, no longer can. This is common, as bodies change. Pelvic floor therapy is available in nearly every major city, and covered by most types of insurance.

If any of the following symptoms or conditions are troubling you, pelvic floor therapy may offer a solution:

- Pelvic pain
- Incontinence
- Hemorrhoids
- Endometriosis
- Recent surgery
- Pain during sex
- Pain in the anus
- Interstitial cystitis
- Recurrent bladder infections

Action Steps

1. Consider mindfulness, purification, diet, and fitness from all episodes prior to this one—feed the *essence*. Practice each routinely.
2. Address burnout with rest, self-care, and renewal—prioritize pleasure in your life. Write in your journal one pleasurable act per day—like catching the sunset.
3. See a doctor or specialist to help balance hormones.
4. Visit a pelvic floor therapist to optimize your sexual response and pleasure.
5. Create romance and schedule time for sex—even with yourself. Add soft music and candles to a hot bubble bath.

Listen to your body and intuition. Become conscious of toxic patterns in relationships, including the one with yourself. Explore healthy ways to release anger and resentment. Practice self forgiveness. Accept yourself. These action steps are exercises to help you regain your essence and joy.

In Conclusion

The CARE Plan for Sexuality and Essence

- Renews sexuality and desire
- Reclaims emotional spark, meaningful connections, novel experiences, and creative explorations
- Prescribes self-care as the key to maintain your sexuality and desire

Revolutionary Beauty Dr. Kathlyn Hendricks, PhD

Dr. Kathlyn Hendricks, PhD is a dancer, internationally known speaker and seminar leader, and trailblazing best-selling author. Dr. Hendricks is the coauthor of the books *Conscious Loving* and *Conscious Loving Ever After* with her husband of 40 years, Dr. Gay Hendricks. Dr. Hendricks is also the cofounder of the Hendricks Institute. I asked her to talk to me about pleasure—a subject she has studied all her life.

Dr. Hendricks: *Women are taught it's not a good idea to receive. We should be last. To be revolutionary is to learn to say, "my turn." Often we resist receiving in unconscious ways. We push away compliments, and we speak negatively about ourselves. The turning point is to say, today I am gong to appreciate myself and find my own beauty.*

*People are more afraid of pleasure than anything. Pleasure is really savoring the joy of being alive, as well as sensory experiences. My sense is we have 2000 years of, "**Oh no!** This is bad, wrong, scary, dangerous," inside us. All the mythologies about women, back to the Garden of Eden promote the message, "Pleasure is dangerous. If women are the source of pleasure, and you can't control them, you have to stifle them. You have to kill them." It sounds dramatic, but this dynamic pervades, the world over.*

William Blake says, "Energy is eternal delight."

For a lot of people, that is triggering. I tell my students, if you don't experience delight, something is blocking it. I get pleasure from experiencing my breath and noticing the play of light. People don't let themselves have pleasure. They don't know how to ride those waves of energy which have been declared bad and wrong. And, we are so afraid of what is going to happen when we feel pleasure. We have genetic memory of terrible things happening to our ancestral grandmothers, midwives, witches, herbalists, and healers—all people who enabled others to enjoy pleasure.

Power has always been on one end, with pleasure on the other. Most people get their juice from power instead of pleasure. That is fear based. That is how I see those two related. The pleasure center is located in our pelvis. We've been taught to disconnect from that. It's time for women to change that and rediscover pleasure—but not as something related to anyone else, just ourselves.

Creativity sparks pleasure. It's the foundation of passion in a long relationship—that and autonomy. Gay and I are completely connected, but autonomous. He is not responsible for my joy, though he is often a source of my joy. We think of pleasure as kind of nasty, but to let purpose flow through me. I am here, not to serve others, but to let purpose flow through me. Gay says I have an amazing shimmer now!

The feeling of being on fire with creativity is revolutionary— and creativity and pleasure dance together.

MODULE 7

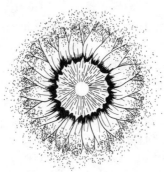

Episode 14
LET IT GLOW!

"Aging is a fact of life. Looking your age is not!"
—Dr. Howard Murad, MD, Antiaging Pioneer

The skin shows the world our level of vibrancy, receptivity, and lust for life. We want to glow. If you want to lift years from your face, an abundance of choices are yours.

In a book about beauty, you may wonder why skin care is covered in "Module 7," rather than at the beginning. Ninety percent of the skin's smooth sparkle depends on what transpires inside the body. Purification practices such as lymphatic drainage, colon cleaning, and fasting are the skin's best friend. The skin, known as the *third kidney*, is a key filtration system. Cleansing is vital to the skin's radiance and well-being. Due to constant toxic exposures, as well as stress, the skin must work overtime to cleanse the cells.

Gorgeous skin, like a joyful attitude and strong body, does not come in a bottle. The effort to cleanse, protect, and pamper the soul's beautiful covering, grants priceless rewards.

Uppermost is saving a bundle on beauty protocols. Puffy skin and cellulite, skin irritations, fine lines, and wrinkles are generally healed with natural solutions. Women spend billions of dollars annually on products to disguise health issues that affect the skin. Yet, few are truly regenerative.

The Queen of Natural Living, Patricia Bragg, applies nothing to her face except organic olive oil and a smile. While a few fine lines are visible, no wrinkles grace her face. Though Patricia scorns anything unnatural, some of us are not blessed with her history. Most people have not feasted on a lifetime of organic food or gallons of vegetable juice and fasted regularly. Those rituals, plus her perpetual spunk, are the foundation Patricia's flawless complexion.

Few things in life are black and white. How we each choose to celebrate and embrace age is unique and personal. *Celebrate* may mean botox or a facelift to one woman. To another, *embrace* may include the choice *not to* color gray hair or eradicate crow's feet. We honor whatever path you choose. Revolutionary Beauties please themselves—that is what defines them as revolutionary.

Dr. Julia T. Hunter, MD, world-renowned dermatologist and longevity expert, teaches that success of any skin technique is dependent on how you care for your skin daily—as well as your mind and body.

Dr. Hunter encourages focus on these three essentials:

1. Stress reduction
2. Sleep
3. Self-acceptance

Stress Reduction

Stress reduction is key to skin that glows. Tension is immediately revealed—whether through blemishes, frown lines, or a dull, lifeless pallor. One of my clients, Janine, reported that she never breaks her daily appointment to practice slow, diaphragmatic breathing. She considers this a beauty ritual, as well as a mental energy balm. Elisabeth swears her weekly 24-hour fasts are what built her ageless beauty. New acquaintances gasp when they hear she is 65, rather than 45. When asked, Elaine whispers that her beauty secret is solo time in an infrared sauna.

Deborah loves 10 to 15 minute power naps. This stops the stress from building throughout the day and resets mood. *Talk about renewable energy.*

What is Patricia Bragg's beauty secret for her skin? Apple cider vinegar, of course! Pour a cup or two into a bath and soak for at least twenty minutes. This regenerative ritual relaxes your mind and muscles, while purifying the skin.

Epsom salt baths are also excellent. Instead of pouring Epsom salt directly into your bath, wet your hands and scoop some of the salt into them. Then, rub your body gently with the salt. Exfoliate your skin. Within a few minutes, your skin will feel tingly with a baby soft quality.

In the heat of a particularly stressful time, refer to the meditation and journaling exercises in "Module 1." Practice daily to de-stress. Highly stressful episodes can age the skin five years in five weeks. When life is skipping along smoothly—or when it takes a dramatic turn—we tend to ignore self-care.

While working with trauma survivors, I designed a tool for healing, *The Lifeline List.* This self-created list highlights health practices which expediently renew you during a crisis. These are the tools we commonly forget when panic, anxiety, and fight or flight take over. My Lifeline List is scanned into my phone and pinned on my closet door.

We suggest you write your own. Do not forget anything—even simple rituals such as:

- Hydrating
- Moving every hour
- Taking supplements
- Monitoring your blood sugar
- Eating healthy meals (three times a day)
- Most importantly, seven to eight hours of sleep

They Call it "Beauty Sleep" for a Reason

Sleep deprivation takes an enormous toll on the skin. This is why evening repose is aptly called *beauty sleep*. How many of us receive the sleep our bodies need? Lack of sleep is high on the list of serious health issues for women. Though stress is the most common contributing factor to insomnia, hormone imbalance affects this condition as well. One can negatively trigger the other. When we do not sleep enough, elevated levels of the stress hormone, cortisol, are produced. Higher cortisol leads to increased stress and inflammation. Lack of sleep also causes a breakdown of collagen and hyaluronic acid—two key ingredients which give the skin a radiant glow.

If you have trouble sleeping, consider the practice of meditation as a daily ritual. Simple, engaging online programs and phone apps that aid mindfulness are plentiful. These programs feature *brain games* that assist the release of stress and anxiety. Additionally, they are fantastic for pain reduction. While recovering from ankle surgery, I used a phone app called HeartMath that measured my heart rate and focused my breathing. My pain was reduced by 75 percent.

Though many countries cherish the afternoon nap or siesta, closing one's eyes in the middle of the day is anathema in America. In fact, many of us feel shame if we are not working in our spare time—let alone napping. No wonder we're exhausted, frazzled, and burned-out. Napping is an incredible gift of renewal to the mind and body. If you need permission to unplug, tune out, and surrender—go right ahead!

American Beauty—Forever 21

The truth is, no plastic surgeon can make dull lifeless skin sparkle. Botox and fillers decrease the appearance of lines. However, if the skin is not thick and resilient, the result can look like a tight caricature of one's self. We have all seen sad pictures of movie stars whose beauty quest has gone wrong.

How does this happen? The pressure of looking 21 forever escapes no one in this youth worshipping culture. Yet, we want to feel and look beautiful. With this program, our intention is that you feel so comfortable in your skin that your choices reflect self-love and acceptance. Let's liberate ourselves from the angst of competition. Today, let's sever ties from a perfectionist beauty model that denies individuality.

The phrase *face value* describes society's definition of superficial beauty. Women have been taught since birth to believe that value is based on physical allure. Society is unforgiving. We have seen extraordinarily strong women succumb to this narrow vision of beauty. For decades, with few exceptions, the only Brown and Black women on the silver screen or in fashion magazines were light skinned, *café au lait* beauties with European features. The standards for American beauty parallel the unhealthy, unnatural Standard American Diet. This model does not support the assertion that each woman is uniquely beautiful—no matter the shape of her eyes or nose, skin pigment, or the number of years she has graced this earth.

This module is a mandate to reinvent and redesign the image of beauty. Beauty itself is a neutral term that stands for the purity and elegance of Mother Nature's creations. As a teenager, without hair or eyebrows (medication side-effects),

I rebelled against the *Barbie Doll* image. I wore Bohemian gypsy dresses and hiking boots. For years, I clung to the role of *righteous rebel*—only to discover that persona was born of insecurity and fear, as much as it grew from the spirit of independence.

Research shows that our internal beauty image was shaped in childhood and teen years—when we were most suscep-tible to societal and cultural beliefs. Who was not insecure in their teens? This alone tells us something about the beau-ty-wound we carry. Regardless, we can shift our self-image to reflect a present state of strength, joy, and self-accep-tance. What is the most attractive, irresistible quality a per-son may possess? Confidence.

Of course, gorgeous, youthful skin equals ageless beauty. In the next few episodes, you will learn about products and simple practices that rewind time for your skin.

In Conclusion

The skin performs many critical functions—regulating tem-perature, synthesizing Vitamin D from the sun, and aiding immunity. When we focus on skin health, the reward is a ro-bust immune system, as well as a youthful glow.

Fanatical dietary habits or an ascetic lifestyle are unneces-sary to renew the skin. In fact, obsessive practices can cre-ate stress that undermines joy and playfulness. Savor an occasional glass of wine and celebratory feast, guilt-free. As Revolutionary Beauties, we are dedicated to pleasure and choice in all forms—including skin care.

Action Steps

1. Return to "Module 1" and choose your go-to healthy stress reducers—whether journaling, bouncing on a rebounder, or meditating.

2. Create a *Lifeline List*. That is a list you create to high-light the health practices that most expediently re-new you during a crisis. This may include aromather-apy massage (one of my favorites), deep breathing, yoga, or the elliptical machine.
3. Personalize the list by coloring, doodling, or collag-ing. Then, hang it on the back of your bathroom or closet door. Photograph it and keep on your phone or use as a screensaver on your computer.

Revolutionary Beauty Malea Rose

Actress, writer, and founder of Vie En Rose Beauty Skincare Line, Malea Rose, shares her story of growing up as a "Bragg Baby" and how that influenced her decision to start her own natural skincare line.

Malea: *I was born and raised on the north shore of Kauai—it has a pure soul. Growing up there was like living in the spirit of the 1970s. Between the landscape and my mom and her hip-pie-goddess girlfriends, I was in awe of it. My mom came from New York City, and she was so ahead of her time. She wanted to live in nature with like-minded men and women in an open-hearted community. When my mom got to Kauai, she realized there was no organic food. We didn't have boutique health food stores; everything had to be shipped in. People were not so aware of what they were putting in their bodies, as they are today.*

My mom started the first co-op on Kauai, and it was all Bragg products—everything was Bragg. It's been engraved in me, seeing Patricia's face on the bottles of the foods I ate as a child.

I grew up as a vegan; I thought carob was chocolate. My mom would make me mac n' cheese with soy cheese. In those days, there were no natural skincare products, and my mom was washing her face with Dr. Bronner's and putting coconut oil on her skin. I grew up on Bragg and still put Bragg's Liquid

Aminos on everything, whether it's Chinese or Italian. Bragg was a part of my life, we bought all the products. I had no idea how much extra love and nourishment I was getting and how ahead of her time she was. That's why I get so starstruck by Patricia Bragg, because I know what she built and what she represents. I get it!

I was a competitive surfer and yet, growing up on Kaui, I didn't feel beautiful. I wasn't the ideal. There at that time, beauty meant dark skin and light eyes. It was about being a local girl and I was not. I am still that same freckly insecure little girl.

Now, I feel beauty is when there is something that emanates from you that catches someone's eye. Beauty is an essence. I think growing up where my life was not centered around material things to make me happy, made me who I am. The values were about being very grounded as a person, making genuine friends, and being real. Kauai still humbles me, my mother humbles me. I have learned life is about being willing to put in the work, to finish things you begin. I like to work hard, I like to see things come to fruition. I am so passionate that when I care about it I have tunnel vision. And, hard work doesn't scare me.

I have been mixing my own skincare products forever, using rich, organic oils, and essential oils, trying to figure out what would work for my skin. At the end of the day, all of our chemistry is different. I have never been able to find a skincare line that makes up for dehydration. When I began acting, I discovered that I would get breakouts from the skincare and makeup.

When I moved to Los Angeles from Kaui, I was used to clean, fresh air. All of a sudden, I was working on sets with nonstop makeup and powder, and they cake it on again and again, and it was absorbing right into my face. I began making my own potions and lotions. I had terrible rashes from allergies and I couldn't find anything. I love acting, but I hated waiting on other people. That was so hard. I have never been able to sit around and wait for something to happen! I don't want my source of happiness to be in other people's hands. The women I was playing in films were stereotyped, they were not empowered women; they weren't as smart as I'd like to portray women. I want to have something that I am passionate about that is my baby. Every color, smell, ingredient, artwork, every element is mine, and it's so exciting to see it come to fruition. The trials and tribulations of one's own product.

I began making potions for my friends, and when it comes to beauty from within, what is better than seeing your best friends feel beautiful? Now, I can do that on a macro level. It's beauty, health, wellness, along with the benefits of cannabidiol (CBD), and I can share that with the world. This is grass roots—I am the janitor, designer, formulator (with my lab). I designed every piece, choosing this shade of pink. The butterflies on the boxes represent the process we all go through—the metamorphosis. They represent growth and power.

My company has been formed by women entirely. I have outsourced to women from Serbia to Berlin, and made friends in the process. The women who work in packaging, now they are women I've called to consult. Everyone has been gracious and wonderful, but the bottom line is, this is my vision.

I am so happy to bring CBD to the world. Not only are these products antiaging, they make you happy. I think stress, sadness, and pain rob us of beauty. I wake up and take ten minutes to think of what I'm grateful for. I say positive affirmations, and visualize having a fabulous day. A lot of my self-care is caring for my body and mind. If I'm going to eat that bag of cookies, you're going to see it on my face as a breakout. Stress eating is a disaster. My beauty ritual is self-love. Smiling is wonderful.

When I told my mom that you asked me to be part of this, she said, "Yay, me!" Yeah, yay, you! Mom, you did it! You raised a Bragg Baby, and here I am, taking that message out into the world. Clean beauty is so important. I've been idolizing the attention to detail that Bragg has always used. There's a video of her online talking about olive oil and how she puts olive oil on her skin; she has so much passion, elegance, grace, strength, and power.

In her era, people weren't talking about DIY. Same with food, nobody knew. Young people are now willing to spend more for their health and organic products. People must have thought Paul Bragg was crazy. He and Patricia were so far ahead of their time. How incredible of Patricia Bragg to leave the legacy she is, it's all about joy and it emanates from her. I think she's so good and she's so infectious and so powerful because she's so **passionate!** She's not bullshitting you, she lives and breathes it. **She's real.**

And, I am in a business that I genuinely love. My goal is to bring clean beauty to the world, beauty from the inside out. Isn't that what it's really about?

MODULE 7

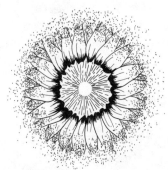

Episode 15
LET IT HEAL: SKIN CONDITIONS

"Your skin is the fingerprint of what is going on inside your body, and all skin conditions—from psoriasis to acne to aging—are manifestations of your body's internal needs."

—Dr. Georgianna Donadio, MSc, DC, PhD,
Nightingale Scholar, Nurse, Chiropractor, and Visionary

Effective, natural solutions to most skin conditions are possible. "Band-aid cures," frequently given by well-intentioned professionals, temporarily repress symptoms. Yet, they do not treat underlying causes. Baffled by protocols devoid of long-term results, I asked a number of skin experts how they determine a patient's course of action. The answer was unanimous. "We believe most patients prefer a quick fix!"

You will find the best care if you entrust yourself to a holistic dermatologist who focuses on the whole body—and desires responsible, committed patients. Beautiful skin can be yours through patience and consistency. In this episode, we share simple rituals that renew skin and do not cost *a queen's ransom*. Turn your home into a spa and pamper yourself. While some skin enhancements require a professional touch, you can peel years from your face (literally) in your home spa. When you find a doctor whom you trust, keep those twice-a-year skin check visits. Any type of skin cancer caught early is immensely more treatable.

Puffy Skin and Cellulite

Puffy skin and cellulite are caused by toxins trapped in lymphatic tissue. Though these glue-like lumps and bumps seem permanent, you are not stuck with them. They respond well to diet changes, fasting, and lymphatic drainage therapy, which you can do at home. If *cottage cheese skin* is the reason you haven't been in a bathing suit for a while, take heart. Reach for your dry skin brush, get your bounce on with a rebounder, and consider seeing a professional lymphatic therapist. These formulas work. We've seen stubborn cases of cellulite clear completely. And, since cellulite signals an inflammatory issue in the body, when you heal it naturally, you strengthen your immune system and boost your energy. You'll not only look great, but feel great.

Rashes and Skin Irritations

Skin rashes almost always signal a systemic issue. Rashes and irritations are often caused by allergies—whether to a food, an animal, a metal, fabric, detergent, or an ingredient in a topical cream. Your doctor can order allergy tests for you, and while they are not 100 percent accurate, they can be an excellent place to start.

Food allergies begin in the gut. If we are not digesting food, it doesn't get assimilated by the small intestine. In fact, it is not recognized as food, but as a foreign substance—a toxin. The immune system attacks that toxin, to which we develop an allergy. When the immune system is overwhelmed by a multitude of these toxins, we begin to develop random allergies. Allergies are seen first as skin rashes before they evolve into more serious symptoms—asthma, chronic headaches, inflammation, and gut disorders such as irritable bowel syndrome (IBS) and colitis. However, none of these are life sentences. Don't let any doctor or health professional tell you that you are, "just going to have to live with it." Patricia Bragg would have some *fighting words* for anyone who would say such a thing.

If you are plagued with sugar or carbohydrate cravings as well as a rash, the cause is likely yeast overgrowth or candida. This can be the result of antibiotic therapy, or too much sugar, carbohydrates, and alcohol, as discussed in earlier in "Module 4." Stress can also trigger candida, as it disrupts the pH in the gut. The permanent fix is diet change and herbal formulas. This combination will also reduce or eliminate sugar and carbohydrate cravings, bloat, and vaginal yeast infections that accompany systemic candida. For more information, see the Resource Guide for suggested herbs.

Contact dermatitis is another cause of skin irritations. Just as the name implies, it's caused by the skin coming into contact with certain substances that some find toxic. Common allergens are nickel, often used for costume jewelry, preservatives in processed foods and topical creams, certain fragrances, and man-made fabrics as well as some natural fibers such as wool. Again, medical tests can determine which specific products and materials create an allergic reaction.

Staph is another common infection that can cause rashes. Antibiotics may be effective, and necessary, if the infection is due to a cut or acute condition. Yet, they do not always *cure* the infection. I have known thousands of clients who experienced temporary relief from antibiotics, only to experience a staph recurrence a few weeks or months later. Detoxification and purification are key to healing—especially after a course of antibiotics. If you are affected by recurrent skin issues, check your thyroid. A colleague, a functional medicine doctor, says that in each case of chronic staph he has seen, a sluggish thyroid is the issue. If you have been diagnosed with chronic staph, contact a medical professional who can advise you on the severity of your staph infection, and options for natural remedies to heal your staph, plus your thyroid and immune system.

Fine Lines and Wrinkles

To reduce fine lines and wrinkles, Patricia Bragg would say, "Drink water and use more olive oil!" And, she would be right. Hydration and a weekly full body oil massage (even one we give ourselves) goes a long way towards plumping the skin. Dehydration is the skin's biggest enemy. While oil and water may not mix, we need them both. Be sure to include plenty of sugar-free coconut water or electrolytes in your drinking water to boost your body's assimilation of fluids. Many clients suffering chronic dehydration were indeed drinking plenty of water, but before electrolyte supplementation, they were *peeing it out.*

Balancing hormones also promotes skin regeneration, especially as we age. Hormone supplementation, whether bioidentical or herbal, supports collagen renewal and keeps the skin from developing spots and discolorations. As you read in "Module 6," many options for balancing hormones are offered. All of them positively affect the skin.

As for skin elasticity, genetics play a role. If your mother, aunts, and grandmother developed bags under their eyes by 40, and you are noticing the same, minor surgery may be the only permanent solution to eliminate them. If so, Dr. Hunter says this procedure has little downtime, and can change your outlook on life. An expert dermatologist can tell you if your skin issue falls into this category.

Ask your dermatologist or aesthetician about professional peels, an excellent solution for fine lines and wrinkles. Deep peels utilize fruit acids to remove the top layers of the skin, which reveal the soft unmarked layers below. Peels remove dead skin cells and stimulate collagen production. As the skin heals post-peel, white blood cells rise to the surface, which plump, soften, and brighten the skin. However, peels require downtime as the skin scabs and heals. Plan ahead, at least a week or two before a special event. We suggest deep peels be administered only by professionals. Nevertheless, you can try gentle peels regularly in the privacy of your own home.

To heal decades of sun damaged skin, Dr. Hunter recommended that I undergo a professional peel. However, I did not book any downtime. The next day, my face looked like I had sunbathed in the Sahara Desert. Immediately contacting the clients I had booked the morning after, I warned them not to faint when they saw me. Luckily, the first lovely lady who appeared at my office door exclaimed, "Oh, you had a peel! You'll be so happy in about a week."

She was right. My skin was renewed. Fine lines and deep wrinkles disappeared. Though a series of peels may be required to achieve desired results, they do work. What a mood lift.

If your best friend or partner is wondering what to get you for your birthday, suggest a consult with a skin professional. This may include a peel or other facial treatment. Since all skin is different, a knowledgeable guide is imperative. Book your appointment with a medical office or spa that offers natural, toxin and cruelty-free products.

Acupuncture facelifts are becoming more common and accessible. I can attest to the reduction of fine lines which lasted months after my first acupuncture facial. The practitioner used no topical creams, potions, steams, or extractions—only strategically placed tiny acupuncture needles. Originating from eastern medicine, this ancient art and science embraces the holistic body. Stimulating facial points with these needles reduces wrinkles as well as refreshes your organs. These tiny needles are not painful.

Enemy #1: Protect Yourself from UV Light

The avoidance of exposure to strong ultraviolet (UV) light—including sunlight—is critical for healthy skin care. Basal cell and squamous cell skin cancer have been linked to UV light. As much as we love to sunbathe, UV light causes wrinkles by damaging the top collagen layer known as the *dermis*.

Before you make a date with the sun, grab a hat and scarf, even for an early morning or late afternoon romp. UV light is present in both foggy and clear conditions. Skin block is essential. Choose a nontoxic sunblock that does not contain paraben or other harmful chemicals. Zinc and titanium oxide are safe alternatives to conventional sunblocks that contain chemicals. These toxins are literally *cooked* into the skin during sun exposure. See Dr. Julia Hunter's website in the Resource Guide for safe UV protection.

Action Steps

Ponder these questions and write the answers in a journal:

- What is my unique asset?
- What do I love about myself?
- What do I want to change, and why?
- For whom do I want to feel beautiful?
- Is it safe to be beautiful? And if not, why?
- Do I give myself permission to feel beautiful?
- What does beauty and radiance mean to me?

I trust your answer to the last two questions is, "Me!" In this spirit, let's learn the secrets of glowing skin, to turn back the clock and boost your confidence.

Revolutionary Beauty Dr. Julia T. Hunter, MD

Meet Harvard trained Dr. Julia T. Hunter, MD, internationally known dermatologist, and founder of Wholistic Dermatology in Beverly Hills, California. Dr. Hunter addresses the body *as a whole*—from inside and out, optimizing skin, and body health. An authority on physiologically correct peels, skin products, bioidentical hormones, and what works and why, she is a noted speaker on the healthiest, best alternatives for maximizing and maintaining health and beauty. Dr. Hunter provides pragmatic, result oriented solutions in treating acne, aging, and skin diseases, promoting skin restoration and prevention for men, women, and teens.

Dr. Hunter has been my dermatologist for a decade. Her three-decade submersion in the field of alternative medicine, studying with leaders and mentors worldwide to expand her knowledge of alternatives to toxic and inflammatory practices and products, has given her an extraordinary toolbox. Her in-depth knowledge has also fueled her belief that the Bragg Healthy Lifestyle is key to both health *and* beauty.

Dr. Hunter: *The number one beauty secret is, "Be healthy and happy!" I can't make a miracle happen with someone's skin if they are not healthy; or if they're miserable.*

Nothing I can do will fix that—no laser in the world makes someone's eyes sparkle. You have to do that on your own. You're the captain of your own ship. Don't forget that. Being beautiful is about energy. What do people see when they look at your face? Your eyes. They see joy and sparkle in your smile, your sense of humor, which is imperative in managing stress. If you're unhappy, do whatever you can to change that. Life is short. Find what you love and do it.

My motto is, "You are what you eat, food is your medicine and eat right for your blood type." Eat fresh, organic food, lots of greens, and more greens, green juices, green powders.

Get plenty of protein. Drink water, stay hydrated. Your skin is a reflection of what's going on inside. Period.

Julia: Are vitamins and supplements necessary, or can we get everything we need through our food?

Dr. Hunter: *Am I a million times sure that vitamins slow down the clock? Yes, I am. Vitamins and supplements reduce inflammation. Supplements support us; everyone needs them. Good ones mitigate our bad habits, those times we're not eating what we're supposed to. People who take antioxidants, they absolutely age slower and have glowing skin, less skin cancer, and fewer health issues in general.*

Exercise is key. Your skin is a reflection of what's going on inside. I can look at someone's skin and have great insight as to how they eat, if they exercise, if their gut is healthy, and how quickly they are aging.

Gut health is crucial; your health is dependent on having a healthy gut. If your digestion is off, everything is off, including your skin. Forget about spending your hard-earned money on products for your face if your gut is a mess. Make sure you're regular—going to the bathroom at least once a day, but ideally twice. If you have gas and bloating, something is wrong. Gut issues lead to inflammation, and inflammation is the cause of all disease, and it's also the real source of aging. Your lymphatic system needs focus, because it regulates inflammation. It's one of the most important systems in your body, and one that most people, and most doctors neglect. Make sure you're doing your lymphatic drainage, colon cleansing, all of that, because that directly effects your health, your longevity, and the lines on your face.

Julia: What do you recommend to support menopause?

Dr. Hunter: *If people are optimized internally, they're more likely to go through menopause later, which is better for your* skin and brain. Menopause isn't a big deal if you know how to handle it, which is with nutrition, antioxidants, curcumin, Vitamin D, and bioidentical hormones, for men and women. Melatonin is great for preventing breast cancer, and I highly recommend women take it daily.

If you're not taking hormones any longer, in my opinion, supplementation not only slows the aging process, but supports your skin, bones, and brain. Hormones are what feed and renew all three of those, especially the bones and skin; otherwise, they get thin. When the skin loses all its collagen, you're prone to bruising and brown spots. Brown spots are a flag that you need more anti-inflammatory, antioxidant supplements. We're living longer than any past generation; we're antiques. Antiques need to be polished and cared for. We want to feel as vital at 75 and 80 as we do at 40 or 50. Hormones keep our brain sharp and lift our mood. Young people have that massive hormone supply to thank for their resilience and optimism. We can duplicate it, but we have to work at it.

Sleep is critical. We all need to sleep—seven hours at least. Without enough sleep, we are not releasing the stress we're accumulating, and stress is the number one cause of inflammation. Stress also contributes to low thyroid, which ages you even more. Sleep is where repair happens. You can't get by without it. Make sure you're nourishing your adrenal glands with rest, but also supplements. If you're burned-out, they're stressed. Adrenal supplements can be game changers, for mood, energy, and immune health. Also, don't stop exercising—even kids need excercise!

Julia: How we we turn the clock back for our skin?

Dr. Hunter: Use only nontoxic skin products. Don't put anything inflammatory on your skin; that is the largest organ of your body. You can look 20 years younger through diet, detoxification, proper skin care, and healthy supplementation.

Life is an inflammatory event, and inflammation is the cause of all disease. **Go nontoxic!** *Buy only products that do not have inflammatory chemicals. Organic does not mean therapeutic, but nontoxic is better than toxic. As you progress into your thirties you need to start using effective topicals on your skin. The earlier a woman starts taking care of her skin, the better.*

Julia: I did not put a thing on my face except olive oil until I was almost 50! And, I spent my life in the sun.

Dr. Hunter: *And, you had the sun damage to show for it, haha. That's why you had to do all those peels, which I'll talk about soon.*

The most important thing for skin is Vitamin C, internally and externally. Vitamin C, when it's present in high concentration in the skin, forces new collagen, gets rid of fine lines, lifts, and adds volume. Currently, people in their early thirties are aging more quickly due to the toxins in the environment, and the enormous stress they carry. I am finding with all my patients in their thirties, their thyroid is more likely to be low. I always recommend an iodine supplement for support and balance.

Next, you need retinol and retinoic. There are a lot of retinols out there, and a lot of different Vitamin Cs. The thing is, Vitamin C is a water soluble vitamin, so if you're using a liquid, you may not be getting anything. Even liposomal packets lose their potency. That's why I created a powder. My Vitamin C powder for the skin is stabilized in glutathione, which is the strongest antioxidant after melatonin. I highly recommend glutathione internally and externally; it's key for supporting the body's channels of detoxification. We live in a toxic world, and need to enthusiastically support the body's ability to dump as much of it as possible.

After Vitamin C, add a strong serum as the next step to your skincare. The serum is like a food truck that feeds the skin, just like eating good food nourishes your body. It's so powerful that patients who have shingle outbreaks get immediate relief with my skin serum mixed with lavender oil. It works like a charm. Then, ice the cake with other things, such as topical Vitamin A, which is a retinoid. Make sure the retinoid and Vitamin A you use is stable; most products are not stabilized, and that's the biggest problem for the public. "What is the stabilizer?" Ask that question. Glutathione is the most dependable one.

And, if you wonder whether your products are working, if you don't see the results, it's not happening. You have to see it work to know it's happening. And, don't forget your bones. Aging is not just about the skin; our bones are thinning. I am a huge fan of the mineral Strontium. You have to keep your bones thick and volumized so your skin doesn't sag and fall to the ground. Tightening, lifting, and volumizing is not just about fixing the skin.

Julia: If we do all of this, what can we expect? Can we really turn back the clock?

Dr. Hunter: If you do all of these things, you can look 20 years younger, absolutely. Not 30 years, or 40 years, but definitely 20. That's my goal with every patient, to educate them so they have all they need to get healthy and start turning back the clock.

I can't say this enough: number one, get healthy. And, remember that it's not only about how you look that makes you appear younger, it's having a brain that is 20 years younger. What do people see when they look at your face? Your energy level, the shine in your eyes, your sense of humor. If you're unhappy, change it. Unhappiness leads to stress; stress leads to inflammation, which leads to aging. Stress kills—we know that. People have to seek happiness like a heat seeking missile. And women, stop worrying about every little thing that you don't love about your body! Men don't see your mole, or your cellulite; they see your eyes and your brain, and they don't see things women obsess over.

As we get older, or go down the path of life, as I like to say, there are tools in the toolbox for looking younger. if you are using good quality skin products, eating right, cleansing your body regularly, then you don't need them, but they exist.

Number one is peels. Now, peels can be toxic, so make sure the peel you're using is clean, and if you're getting a professional peel, grill your doctor or aesthetician and ask them what's in their products.

Julia: You suggested I do peels as my skin was damaged, and I had spots that you cautioned could turn into skin cancer.

Dr. Hunter: *Exactly! Peels not only reduce and eliminate those spots, but fine lines. They force collagen production, and they tighten the skin, so with the right peel, you can look a decade younger with little downtime. Three to six months after a peel should yield even better results than the first month, as the collagen production keeps ramping up. I am a huge fan of peels. Peels volumize; they wind the collagen more tightly; they lift; they get rid of fine lines.*

Next, we go to the things that I call "the icing on the cake, the tools in the toolbox." One is Botox.

Julia: Is Botox safe?

Dr. Hunter: *Yes, it is. I've never had one person react to it—if you do it in low doses. There are doctors out there who overdose people, but it's unnecessary, as a little goes a long way. The only people who react have low thyroid; then they may feel a little like they have the flu after they get it. Botox is a safe, well tested tool. You don't have to do it, but it looks good; it doesn't make you sick. There's no downside.*

There's also fillers made of hyaluronic acid, which your own body produces. Putting a little filler in plumps up the face, because ultimately the bones thin no matter what you do and you get hollow temples. We are losing fat in our face, just as we're acquiring the wisdom to know how to live our lives. This is especially true for thin people. Threads are excellent; they lift, tighten, and volumize. So, when reaching into my toolbox, I go for Botox, fillers, and threads.

I have to look at people and evaluate; what serves them best? What is the least obtrusive? What lasts longest? No one ever wants to look as if they've had work done. Technology, in the form of lasers, can be wonderful. Some require no downtime and others do. A note to people with melasma: If people have melasma, they are inflamed internally. They need gut help and anti-inflammatories. Something is wrong if you have melasma; do not try to just fix this with topicals. And never do lasers; they not good for melasma. They make it worse.

On the tech side, InMode lasers are the strongest ones on the market and they do necessitate some downtime. If my patients can't take downtime, I choose a Forma laser, which lifts and tightens, and no one will know. You won't look like anyone did anything. You just look younger and well-rested. The results are fantastic.

I am also a fan of Morpheus, an InMode laser, which requires one week of downtime; it lifts and tightens. It takes nine months to get maximum results from this treatment, as it makes a massive amount of collagen, and keeps making it for a year. In a year, your face has plumped up and out the way it was when you were young. I say, I can see "the girl" in my patient's faces again. I want to see the light in their eyes.

Whatever products you use, you need to put it on your eyelids, face, neck, hands. If you don't put skin products on all those places, something will look old! Don't use a product you can't put on your eyelids.

When I use technology, I recommend a strong treatment every couple of years. In the meantime, my patients are doing *self-care, all the good things. Women who have a facelift and haven't cared for their skin, their result will be fleeting. After the inflammation goes away, in a few months, they will be very disappointed with how they look. They did nothing to make collagen; and they can look like skeletons with skin stretched over their skull. It's not a pretty look. It's not soft.*

One thing about compounded drugs; people think compounded drugs are nontoxic. Most compounded drugs and creams are some of the most toxic creams on the market. Research how the products you use are made.

Julia: What should avoid?

Dr. Hunter: *Here's my list:*

- *Avoid not sleeping*
- *Avoid not being happy*
- *Avoid not being healthy*
- *Avoid being constipated*
- *Avoid a laser if you have melasma*
- *Avoid looking like you had work done*
- *Avoid anything that creates inflammation*
- *Avoid thinking there is one solution to everything*
- *Avoid anything toxic—check peels—many are toxic*
- *Get rid of heavy metals through cleansing and use green powder, greens, garlic, onions*

We're watering the flowers, a little of this a little of that; good food, good supplements, good products, happy life. Smell the flowers. Do what you love.

Dr. Hunter created a product line, Skin Therapy. She has a private practice in Beverly Hills, California; London, England; and Geneva, Switzerland. Find her at juliathuntermd.com.

MODULE 7

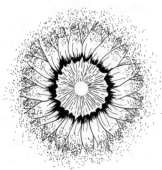

Episode 16
THE 5-MINUTE
CARE SKIN PROGRAM

"Beautiful skin requires a commitment, not a miracle."

—Dr. Erno Laszlo, Skin Care Pioneer—introduced philosophy
of *confidence through healthy skin*

"The CARE Plan" in this module targets five easy steps to
skin preservation and renewal:

1. Gentle cleansing
2. Exfoliate and renew
3. Tone and rebalance
4. Replenish collagen and restore vitamins
5. Hydrate and protect

This effective program takes five minutes a day. Only one
obstacle can successfully sabotage our sense of beauty—to
fall into the trap of the *compete and compare cycle*. We will
never look exactly like the actresses in magazines, as those
pictures are retouched from top to bottom. None of us

parade around with filters and backlights which shine golden tones on our faces. However, we *can* look twenty years younger, and be the *best* version of ourselves. We can eliminate fine lines, tighten the jawline, and reduce wrinkles. When we combine *state of the art* protocols with time-tested, natural products, we reboot collagen production and reverse aging. At 66, my skin looks softer, and my face has fewer lines than a decade ago. So can yours. Every tool I discovered to defy aging is shared within the pages of this book.

Who has more than five minutes, twice a day, to spend on skin care? No woman I know. So, with experts, we created a fast, easy, affordable, and potent program. Let's get to it!

Step One—Gentle Cleansing

Even the most traditional rituals—such as scrubbing faces till squeaky clean—are under scrutiny. We know that harsh soaps age skin. Experts agree that natural, gentle cleansers, and toners are best.

The five types of cleansers are:

1. Oil Cleansers—You may clean your face with oil, especially if your skin is dry. Use a pure, organic oil, such as olive or coconut oil. Consider substituting an oil for a soap cleanser once a week. Avocado and aloe vera gel mixed together is a wonderful, natural oil cleanser.
2. Soap Cleansers—If you enjoy the crisp, clean feel of soap, organic cleansers such as castille are gentle and safe. Castille can be infused with healing essential oils such as lavender or peppermint. Verify that your soap is 100 percent natural and chemical-free. Experts suggest switching cleansers and shampoos every few months to keep skin and hair fresh.
3. Honey Cleansers—Honey naturally regenerates the collagen in skin. You may find honey as an ingredient in many organic cleansers. However, you can whip up

your own honey cleanser by adding a few drops of lemon juice, or apply it right from the honey pot. We are grateful to those amazing bees and the healing properties of honey.

4. Clay Cleanser—Clay is time-consuming cleanser to use daily. Nevertheless, a weekly clay mask tighten and exfoliate the skin as well as stimulate your glow.

5. Micellar Water—Simplify cleansing even further with micellar water—purified water infused cleansers with suspended oil particles known as micelles. Both cleansing and slightly moisturizing, clear micellar waters remove makeup and sweat without stripping the skin of natural oils. Choose micellar water which is free of parabens, sulfates, and alcohol. Some prefer to use micellar water as a makeup remover, followed by a gentle cleanser. While no rinsing is needed after a micellar water cleanse, a cold water rinse makes for a refreshing finish.

Cold Water Rinses

Cold splashes are incredible for the skin and immune system. Warm water opens pores for deep cleaning. Cold water closes them. Rinse your face with cold water as part of your morning and evening rituals. If you feel brave, world renown naturopath, Richard Schulze, PhD, recommends that at the end of a hot shower, switch to a cold spritz for sixty seconds. This instantly reduces inflammation, lowers cortisol, and boosts adrenals. Though common for centuries in Scandinavia, ice baths are becoming popular additions to spas around the world—particularly alternating hot soaks with cold plunges.

Once you try a cold water rinse after a warm shower, you will be hooked. Inspired by "Iceman" Wim Hof, Revolutionary Beauty, Josette Tkacik recently hosted training-in-home ice baths. Find Wim Hof's website in the Resource Guide.

Step Two—Exfoliate and Renew

Daily exfoliation with cleansing grains or mild retinoid transforms your skin over time. Retinoids are derived from a potent form of Vitamin A. Strong exfoliants may be used twice
a week, such as larger cleansing grains or alpha hydroxy fruit
acids. For chemical peels—including fruit acids—visit a professional aesthetician or dermatologist periodically.

Cleansing Grains—Oatmeal is one of the grains that makes
an excellent skin cleanser and exfoliator. Chemical-free oatmeal cleansers—whether homemade or from the health
food store—are gentle on the skin and can be used daily.
Other homemade skin exfoliators include salt-based pastes.

For those of you who prefer a cutting edge approach to
skin exfoliation, dermatologists recommend a retinol based
product. When used topically in high concentrations, this
product causes the skin to peel slightly, exfoliating dead
cells. Collagen boosting retinoids are generally used once or
twice a week to aid skin renewal, sunspot removal, fine lines,
and wrinkles. Retinoids come in many forms, from alpha-be-
ta hydroxy acids to lighter retinals. Your dermatologist or
aesthetician will recommend the best for your skin type.

Alpha and Beta Hydroxy Acids—These compounds are derived from fruit acids and available over-the-counter (OTC).
They are also produced in pharmaceutical-grade dilutions,
administered by a dermatologist. Even a naturally based
fruit acid removes the top layer of skin. This causes a slight
burning of the skin that allows the soft, unmarked layers to
surface. Alpha and beta hydroxy acids create radiant, youth-
ful-looking skin, with diminished fine lines and wrinkles. I dab
a few drops of peel on my face twice a week, alternating
with a dermatologist recommended Retin-A.

Natural OTC products can be used safely at home. However,
if you are sensitive to topical products, test on your forearm

before applying to your face. When in doubt, speak to a dermatologist or aesthetician.

Retinoids—Derived from Vitamin A, these creams come in various strengths. Experts recommend retinoid use begin in the twenties, as it is an excellent remedy for acne. If, instead, you spent your youth slathered in baby oil, baking in the sun, you can still rescue your skin. All retinoids should be used only at night, as they are sun sensitive and sun reactive.

Step Three—Tone and Shine with ACV

Aestheticians recommend a quality toner after cleansing. Toners purge blocked pores and rebalance the pH level of the skin that soaps may strip away. A little known secret is that you can find one of the best, natural toners in your kitchen pantry—apple cider vinegar. And no, you will not smell like vinegar later. Choose a skin toner with a slightly acidic pH, about 5.5. You can use over-the-counter pH strips to test new skin products. Dip a pH strip into a capful of toner to measure acidity. A pH-balancing toner, such as ACV, tightens skin, so be sure to apply to your neck and chest as well as your face.

Step Four—Replenish with Powdered Vitamin C

Vitamin C is the most important element for skin renewal. Mix a pinch of high quality powdered Vitamin C with water. Gently apply to your face every morning after toner. Allow the Vitamin C to dry before moisturizing.

DeeDee Serpa-Wickman, cofounder of Skin Prophecy, discovered the power of Vitamin C decades ago. Her signature organic botanical skin care line was created through DeeDee's and her sister's 28 years of clinical experience as aestheticians. They learned that when applied directly to the skin, natural powdered Vitamin C is one of the most preventative and restorative agents for antiaging and skin care.

"The CARE Skin Program" recommends the daily use of the antioxidant Vitamin C powder to stimulate collagen and tighten the skin. Vitamin C skincare products are found in salons, drugstores, or almost any beauty counter.

As I did not begin a skin care program until my fifties, professional skin care rejuvenation was required to set me on the right path. Though Patricia Bragg swears by olive oil as her beauty secret, some of us need more. Lines and wrinkles that have accumulated for years do not dissolve overnight. Once upon time, products and procedures used by the rich and famous were well hidden secrets. Now, a whole world of innovative, transformative beauty treatments are affordable and accessible to all.

Explore multiple ways to improve elasticity, diminish age spots, reverse sun damage, and *get your glow on* at any age. If you are diligent about a skin care routine with the right protocol and products, you will see exciting results.

Step Five—Hydrate and Protect

Hydrating moisturizers are critical for plump and dewy skin. Choose a formula by skin type. Some moisturizers contain both vitamins and peptides. Peptides are protein building blocks naturally found in the skin. One of the best treatments you can add to your daily routine is a peptide serum.

Your moisturizer of choice may be something as simple as Patricia Bragg's beauty balm, organic olive oil. Essential oils, such as lavender, added to almond oil, is excellent for sensitive, dry skin, or to heal a sunburn. Used alone, lavender oil heals blemishes, cuts, and minor burns. You may also choose a moisturizer with active antiaging properties. Many, like the peptide serum mentioned above, include collagen building properties which restore and restructure skin. Oxygenating serums are superbly effective, and generally oil-free. Oxygen introduced directly into the skin promotes collagen growth.

Hyaluronic acid is deeply moisturizing. Do not let the word "acid" confuse you. Hyaluronic acid adds moisture into the skin by binding water with collagen.

Skin care experts recommend a combination of serums with moisturizers. When you buy products, carefully read ingredients, and follow directions. Choose natural, therapeutic, and chemical-free formulas. As we focus on detoxification practices to eliminate chemicals from our diet and bodies, why apply them to our skin? Since the skin is transparent and porous, that which is applied to the skin, soaks into your body.

A Word About Sunblock

Each morning, apply a natural paraben-free sunblock, even on cloudy days. The habit of applying sunblock daily will protect your skin from UV rays that dry and wrinkle skin, and cause skin cancer. An alternative to the use of sunblock is a hat and scarf, or sun protective clothing.

Many moisturizers contain at least a level 15-30 sunblock. Simplify your skin care routine into a morning ritual that works for you. Follow the five step program for a fast and easy protocol to renew and protect your skin.

During at-home spa days, add a weekly exfoliant. On celebratory visits to your aesthetician, choose a mask or light peel to remove the dead skin. While pampering your face, do not forget the rest of your body. Exfoliating seaweed and salt scrubs deliver silky smooth skin, reduce inflammation, and improve circulation. You will feel wonderful!

Action Steps

1. Simplify your skin care routine to a morning refresh and an evening deep clean, using rejuvenation and restorative hydration. Simply splash your face with cold water in the morning, then follow with a pH balancing

    toner (choose ACV), and hydrating moisturizer with sunscreen. Then, in the evening, carefully remove makeup and grime with a natural cleanser, micellar water, or natural oil. Finally, tone again, add a nourishing serum, and, if your skin is dry, a moisturizer.

2. Try making your own healing skin cleansers, toners, creams, and masks. You don't have to attempt all of them, but find one of the recipes at the back of this book that appeals to you and try.

In Patricia Bragg's youth, the dangers of chemicals to health were almost totally unknown. Women in the 1950s longed to free themselves from the time-consuming labors of their mother's kitchens. They welcomed frozen meals, canned vegetables, and one dish casseroles made with cream of chicken soup. As the famous line from 1960s film, *The Graduate*, predicted, "The future is in plastics."

People thought Paul Bragg and Patricia Bragg were crazy, when each was simply far ahead of their time. Paul introduced radical health protocols and trailblazing practices through lectures and television. Patricia followed spreading the message of health, happiness, and ACV in every country who opened their doors. They created dozens of natural foods and products, and distributed them worldwide. How many women executives of her generation existed, let alone achieved her astounding success?

Patricia Bragg says, "I worked seven days a week and ran my company for 65 years, and not one day of it was work." That is the definition of passion and purpose.

Paul and his feisty, fabulous daughter created a legacy of natural healing and longevity programs from which we all benefit—how lucky we are. Young people are especially appreciative of natural products and protocols. Willing to spend their hard-earned money for health foods, organic produce, and *green packaging*, they understand the value. Years before

I met Patricia Bragg in person, my son, Luke, presented me with a copy of the Bragg's book *Miracle of Fasting* as a Christmas gift. A natural lifestyle devotee, he said, "These were the people that started it all."

Patricia is a testament to clean living. She has danced with grace and joy—never a moment of suffering over her avoidance of alcohol and sugar. No one ever heard her fret about her organic vegan diet. Her daily exercise and meditation was a given. She embraced those practices, and embodied a joy that emanates. Her enthusiasm for physical, mental, and emotional health is infectious, because it is real. She is authentic. She says, "We are what we eat, breathe, think, say, and do."

Following in her footsteps, I am honored to continue her legacy, while attempting to balance those seven-day work weeks. My goal is to extend the Bragg message of health and healing. Like Patricia, this mission launches me from bed each morning, filled with gratitude and fire. There is nothing I would rather do with my wild and precious life.

The desire of the Revolutionary Beauties in this book is to impart to women that aging does not have to be denied or hidden. We also yearn to reach today's youth, who search for a genuine expression of their lives. Patricia Bragg preached, "Live loud, live organic, live happy, and live your own life!" She bravely tossed societal expectations to the wind and said, *"I am beautiful."* That is our wish for you—at any age, in any body, color, shape, or size.

To all of you reading this book—clean deep, glow bright, and change the world. We love you!

—Julia and Patricia

Revolutionary Beauty Erin Elizabeth

Meet trailblazing journalist, Erin Elizabeth, founder of *Health Nut News*. Erin won the Truth in Journalism Award in 2017. She courageously researches health, medicine, and environmental issues. She has spoken to thousands of holistic doctors since 2015. A featured contributor to the series *The Truth About Cancer*, she has been a devotee of the Bragg Healthy Lifestyle all her life.

Erin: *I am excited to be here! I bought Patricia's* Vinegar *book with my babysitting money when I was 14.*

I was born on September 28, 1970, and subsequently put up for adoption. I was very sick, hospitalized for several months right after I was born. I had severe thrush and other health challenges. A few months later I was adopted.

When I was growing up, I was aware that I was much sicker than other kids. Because of my health challenges, I always wondered if there was anything I could do to feel better. At 14, at our local bookstore I came across Paul and Patricia Bragg's Apple Cider Vinegar book. I bought it and I carried it everywhere. They became my heroes. I learned so much reading that book, and quickly became a vegetarian. Luckily, my parents were really supportive. I have that book to this day. When I was a teenager, my family would occasionally go to Hawaii, and I had read about the fitness classes that Paul and Patricia led on Waikiki. I wanted to go. My parents thought it was funny that instead of wanting to go to an arcade or the mall, all I wanted to do was go to those classes.

When I was in high school, a modeling scout saw me. We lived in Chicago. I'm 5'10", and they were interested in signing me. My mom went to New York with me, and I was offered a contract, but it had a caveat—the agency wanted me to lose 20 pounds. I weighed 143, but they wanted me to be 120. I've been 120, and that is way too thin for me. I did do a little runway, and at 143, I didn't fit into the samples. I tried to lose the weight, but I just could not.

So, I went to college, working my way through with a job at Citizen's Action Coalition. I also had a radio show on air, Bringing The Truth to the People. I've always been an activist at heart. But, the rejection I got from that agency over my weight really stung. I carried it with me for a long time. I felt ashamed of my body and my size, even though I look back at pictures of me in those days and think to myself, "Erin, you looked just fine!" I had to learn to accept myself.

I think shame had roots in my childhood, going to a Catholic all-girls boarding school. The nuns were talking about saints who burned themselves to be uglier, as if beauty was a sin. I died my hair funky colors and got in big trouble. They wanted us to be dull and drab. When we think about it, in the animal kingdom, animals show off their beauty, their colors, their coats. Animals groom themselves. I have cats, and they glide across the living room so sassy, as if they're walking on a catwalk. They are divas.

If animals are proud of who they are, why are we dimming our light? I am reminded of a story of another one of my cats. She was ten and had a triple coat. We had her shaved for a skin condition, and she was devastated. The other cat hated her. She smelled different and she was shunned. She got so depressed and stayed that way until her coat grew back. Witnessing that taught me a lot. It's natural to want to be beautiful.

I am always talking about self-care on my blogs because it's so important. I discovered in 2020 when I couldn't get my hair done, or my nails done, what a difference it made in my self-esteem. Now, those are little things, but they make a difference. They make me feel confident. I also tried wearing short hair for a while because I decided I wanted to be low-maintenance. There are taboos about women over 50 having long hair. We're not supposed to want to be sensual or sexy anymore.

But, I have known women who are both of those at 80. Look at Patricia Bragg. She's gorgeous. I also think it's important for women to build up other women. We should complement each other and tear down the stereotype that women compete. The truth is, we want to be collaborative. We want each other's support. We need it.

Julia: Erin, would you share the story of your explant surgery? (Explant is the term for removal of breast implants.) We've learned that breast implants can cause a multitude of health issues, such as chronic fatigue, acute inflammation, and even a hematoma and autoimmune diseases—lupus, RA, and scleroderma.

Erin: *Yes, I would love to. It's such an important topic, and I talk about it publicly whenever I have the chance. I had my saline breast implants removed nine years ago. I got them in my thirties. I had lost weight, and it seemed like my breasts disappeared with my weight loss. I was still doing some modeling part-time, and I think I was still insecure about my looks.*

I learned all about the medical issues that implants can cause, so I decided to have them taken out not that long after I got them. I went to a great surgeon in Atlanta, Susan Kolb, who is an explant specialist. (You can find Susan Kolb on YouTube discussing explant surgery.) It was a six hour surgery. With explants, you want to make sure you go to a reputable surgeon who only does explants, not one who does implants. The procedures are very different.

If you would like your breast implants removed, but you're worried that you might sag, you can ask for a lift and a fat transfer. Suzanne Somers was one of the first women in the United States to use her own fat when she needed implants after cancer surgery. But it's common now. There are explant experts in just about every large city. It's worth the extra time and money to find one, even if you have to sacrifice having that new car for a little while. It's your health.

Somehow, in America, there is this myth that men prefer large breasts. Bigger everything seems to be an American trait. We're taught to covet bigger cars, bigger houses. But I don't believe men care about breast size. My birth mother lived in Europe for nearly 40 years, and I would visit her often. I noticed the French women didn't seem to fret over having small breasts. In fact, they would accentuate that by wearing a tank top. They accentuated the features they loved. If they had great abs, they would wear a midriff blouse. They seemed so comfortable in their skin. It was a cultural confidence and sensuality. I admired it.

What being in Europe taught me was, know your assets. Accentuate your best parts. Love the skin you're in!

Revolutionary Beauty Erin Foster

Meet Revolutionary Beauty Erin Foster, writer, clothing designer for *Favorite Daughter*, which she cofounded with her sisters, Sara and Jordan. She is an advisor to Bumble—a dating app, The Mirror—a home fitness start-up, and Bev—a canned wine company.

Erin married the love of her life, Simon, on New Year's Eve, 2019. She also directed her first music video in the summer of 2020. The daughter of music producer, David Foster, and Dallas born natural beauty, Rebecca Foster, Erin grew up in Los Angeles.

Erin: *I think you set the tone at an early age of how you view yourself. You can have an arrested development at your most insecure point, and that's how you define yourself for the rest of your life. For me, getting attention and feeling beautiful on the outside felt important for so long and I hinged my happiness on what people, especially men, thought of me. I didn't stop to think, "Do I like the person I am?" I just wanted people to like me. I was constantly thinking, "What do they think of me; do they think I'm beautiful?"*

Growing up in Los Angeles and around people who focus so much on beauty, nobody is young enough, hot enough, skinny enough, cool enough, famous enough, or has enough famous friends; it's a never ending need for more. I wanted a lot of those things for a long time. I did compare myself to my sister a lot, because we were so close in age. Things came easy for Sara.

My mom was really wonderful, and it made a huge difference. She's very comfortable getting older; she is at total peace with it, and she always instilled that lack of shame around five extra pounds or lines on your face.

When I was 15, at my most awkward point, overweight, insecure, and self-conscious, my mom and I went shopping for an outfit for my birthday. Nothing was fitting me; I was trying things on—nothing fit. I was in the dressing room, and I heard the sales woman say really loudly, "I think we need a larger size," which I thought everyone in the store could hear. I just fell apart. I started crying and melting down and said, "I hate this, I hate life, and I hate myself!"

My mom said calmly, "Erin, you're 15 years old. This is exactly how you are supposed to feel today. You aren't supposed to peak at 15. You're supposed to peak at 30. You don't want to be perfect today. You have so much more time ahead of you." It took a lot of pressure off of me.

I think I was always negotiating with myself—what's important? What brings me real joy? When do I walk away from a conversation feeling good? I was addicted to flirting and attention and knowing when someone had a crush on me. In my late teens and early twenties, I was always trying to be someone else—a friend or Sara, anything but myself.

It wasn't working; there was a moment or period of time around 26 where I just decided, "I'm going to take a left turn. I'm going to go in a totally different direction. I want to be a comedy writer. Maybe I want to do stand-up. I want to find *friends who watch improv, and who are in tech, or in writing, or journalism. I am going to shift my value system."*

I did that, and I started to feel more like myself. I started writing, and instead of me trying to be this idea of who I thought I should be, I started being honest about who I actually was. I wrote about being rejected, and feeling insecure or having a shame spiral after being on a date when I said the wrong thing. I was scared to date someone nice because they'd find out how broken I was; I'd write anything that was real.

Ironically, when I was becoming my real self on the inside, I started to look different; I started losing weight, and my hair grew long, I stopped dying it red and let it be blonde. I got a lot cuter and I also felt better about who I was. I wasn't trying so hard, and I was blossoming. It felt like I was just becoming who I was meant to be—not to say that I was meant to be skinnier or more attractive, but sometimes we are just carrying so much emotionally that we don't even look like our true selves.

I was always wondering why I was constantly compared to my sister, thinking "it's so unfair, I'll never be her," and I suddenly realized the person who was comparing was me! And, when I adjusted my point of view and changed the narrative, it stopped happening. I found my own personal value system and people stopped comparing us. I found my currency, and my currency was connecting to other women. My currency was being self-deprecating, not for effect, but in a real way. My currency was being vulnerable and being honest, and just being real. And, it really changed what I valued. And, then, my life started to get easier.

Turning 30 was also a beautiful thing. I relaxed, and there was less pressure. I'm not as skinny as I was ten years ago, but I am so much happier. I used to think, "If I could only lose weight, I'd be happier," but now, I'm 15 pounds heavier than I was at my skinniest, and I'm so happy.

I didn't meet my husband until I was 35, and for a long time I was convinced it wasn't going to happen for me. So, I just kind of let go. And, I met someone who sees the best in me. There have been times that I look at my body and think nobody would ever find me beautiful, and in that moment, Simon says, "I have the hottest wife!" And, sometimes it makes me realize that what you see isn't necessarily real. Maybe he's seeing something better, and I'm seeing something worse, but the truth is probably somewhere in the middle, and we trick ourselves into assuming the worst.

I try to be perfect, and sometimes I have to remember a big piece of happiness is letting things go. My biggest struggle is my anxiety and my worry, and I try to do everything fully and efficiently, and I have to give myself a break sometimes and let myself have a glass of wine here and there, even though it's on my list of no's.

I keep the phone far away, and 5G scares me, and I lie on my crystal mat, and I'm so into all of it. That focus can also be an obsession—worrying that everything toxic will kill me—so I am looking for balance, always. But, it's hard to watch people eating food drenched in chemicals. I know what's in junk food and fast-food.

There's a stigma around aging in Los Angeles. My mom is beautiful, and she says her age really proudly. She owns whatever her truth is. I am so grateful I had a mom who proudly turned a new age every year. I'm trying to mimic that.

I think it's important as women to embrace every new phase and chapter, and talk about it openly. Every time a woman embraces her age, it gives permission for someone else to embrace theirs. That's the woman I want to be. It's on us as women to fix this. We allow people to make us feel ashamed of our age. We say it like it's a bad thing. I'm 38 and I wonder, will I freak out when I turn 40? The anxiety is worse than the thing. I'm sure I'll turn 40 and say, "I'm still okay; what's different?"

I think about couples who are envied, and guys who envy their friends' marriage, the people who look at another relationship and say, "I want that." They say that because they want the kind of partner that is making someone happy. They want a partner who sees them and accepts them, and isn't punishing. It's all about being connected to someone and connected to yourself. Being connected to yourself comes first. I loved myself before anyone could fall in love with me.

The more we as women can take the stigma away and be proud of being older, the more we can offer to each other and the world. You have to figure out—what is your voice? What is your voice telling you to say and to do, and go out and take for yourself? You can't do what anyone else is doing. You can't do what your friends are doing. And, if you let yourself be alone long enough, there's a voice that will speak to you—not for attention, not for effect, but when no one is looking and no one can hear it, it will whisper, what do you care about? And, you'll know. And, if you have the means, you have to go after it.

I'm really close to my sisters, both Sara and Jordan. Working with family is challenging, but it's so wonderful to get to do it all together.

Julia: Tell me about the music video you directed?

Erin: *I loved it; it was so fun. I turned down doing it three times. My husband convinced me to do this. He said, "I know you can do this; I'm saying yes." I said, "This is my decision," and he said, "You can't make this decision, you're too afraid, I'm making it for you. Just say yes!" So I did, and I was so happy.*

You have to do things that are a little scary, right?

AFTERWORD

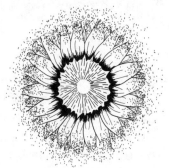

Your Legacy

What does *legacy* mean to you?

To Patricia Bragg, legacy means fulfilling her life's purpose to promote health, and launch a *butterfly effect* of positive change. From a young age, she grasped her mission—to spread the message that health is in our hands. Patricia implores us to create our own positive reality. She commands the world to live clean, avoid chemicals, environmental toxins, and negative thoughts. *The Queen of Natural Living* inspires us to enjoy whole organic food and purify our bodies. She reminds four generations that Mother Nature knows best—and that healing is possible. Millions of lives have been changed by the tenets of the Bragg Healthy Lifestyle.

Those who met Patricia personally, heard her speak on the radio, or saw her on television experienced her sparkle and sass. She preached how Vital Force emanates from living your purpose, living clean, and living large. As spiritual activist Marianne Williamson paraphrased Nelson Mandela, "Your playing small does not serve the world." Everyone who met Patricia has a story—and those stories live on. That is the meaning of legacy. Yet, what does legacy mean to those of us less renowned? What if you have not contemplated anything beyond getting through tough days, hoping you are not forgotten by those who you love, and the knowledge that your life mattered?

Each of our lives do matter. We are all connected. When one of us changes a pattern—leaves a toxic relationship or heals an illness—we send up a flare that attracts the eye of a kindred spirit, who is scanning the horizon for hope. Witnessing a miracle reminds us that miracles happen and they can happen to us. That is the essence of the butterfly effect in action—that many small actions generate enormous impact.

We call this *ordinary magic*. After all, most people who accomplish the extraordinary feats such as those described in this book consider themselves quite ordinary. They are people like us, who, through grit and grace, persevered. We might try multiple ways to climb from what feels like a dark 40-foot well. We seek advice. We take help when offered. But, it is by taking that first step, and then putting one foot in front of the other, that we finally climb out, into the sun. And when we do, the paparazzi are not around to glorify our success. Yet, our journeys do change the world.

That is legacy.

We create legacy through sharing ordinary magic with each other. Women do this constantly, in a thousand languages, in a thousand lands, from bright amethyst dawns to obsidian nights. Some of us whisper stories to each other, in the grocery aisles, at the gym or salon, or at 3 am on the phone. Often, our stories and epiphanies emerge in sacred, solitary time with sips of morning tea, or the momentary spark of a creative project.

When we invite the Spirit and our subconscious to speak to us, to embolden us, to quiet the cacophony of fear just enough, we hear the simple messages that change our lives: "Leave now." "Start now." "You can do this!" "Today is the day."

Whether you scribble notes into a journal or paint color onto a canvas, you open the door to the voice of your truest self. In time, if you listen, those golden messages reveal the blueprint of your unique, exquisite life. The first step is to show up for yourself. Then, take action on what you heard from the small voice of your intuition. Call it Spirit or God, Guides, or Intuition, this voice is available and accessible to everyone. Whether through contemplation, prayer, meditation, or quiet time, showing up for ourselves is the essence of self-care.

Of course, like making green juice and doing push-ups, "showing up" is an action, a verb, not only a noun. In her groundbreaking book, *The Artist's Way*, Julia Cameron teaches a ritual called "Morning Pages," wherein one writes three pages daily, uncensored. This habit nourishes the inner artist and evokes expressive creativity. This creative act requires attention, intention—and then, no tension, as Janet Bray-Attwood wrote in her book, *The Passion Test*. Intention is nothing without attention and action. The tools you have learned in *Revolutionary Beauty* hopefully inspire you to take the next step in your journey to self-care and ageless renewable energy. These practices activate the power to transform your life. Every step is a story—a spark of ordinary magic.

When you share those stories, you create your legacy.

Just as nature is the ultimate healer, she is also the ultimate teacher. Nature teaches self-care, how to create renewable energy through presence and perseverance. A tree reveals a thousand years through rings in its trunk, telling a story of the ages. Yet, the tree has never left the forest. Dig deep into the earth. Inhale the mustiness of her lush fertility. Breathe clean ocean air. Lie on a patch of green. Cultivate wildness.

In nature, beauty is wild, sensual, and free. The pounding current of a river, the vibrancy of a coral reef, reverberate through all of our senses. The irresistible attractions compel our attention. When we become wild again, we are likewise irresistible. We do something bold that we've never done, and to our surprise, we don't die; we fly—we thrive. We tell our story—a story of ordinary magic.

As potent as wild freedom is for the spirit, we require safety to grow roots as well as wings. We need to feel secure to maintain happiness. This precious planet we inhabit is in crisis, as many of us are. As we can heal ourselves, we will heal the world. Nature understands that with the freedom to fly is the expectation—the birthright—of balance and support. Without structure, chaos reigns.

The Laws of Nature are indisputable and unconditional. Nests built on broken branches fall. However, nature offers warnings—the wind shifts before a flood and the earth groans before erupting. *Pay attention*, nature says, and act accordingly. While regeneration is possible following a devastating storm, it is best to heed the warnings of nature. The tired, lifeless look of our reflection in the mirror is Mother Nature's nudging us to take care of ourselves. Create time and space to rest and renew. Sleep and revive in a safe haven that you have built for yourself. Cherish your health so you can thrive. Create a legacy for others to follow and to benefit from what you learned.

I wrote *Revolutionary Beauty* as an homage to Patricia Bragg and the legacy of the Bragg Healthy Lifestyle. These principles rescued me, and saved me from a short life of long hospital stays and needless suffering. Yet, it was through action steps, trial and error, that I healed and transformed my life. My legacy is to offer tools, encouragement, and support. Write me at *revolutionarybeautycrusade@gmail.com* and I will respond. Ask questions and feel free to share your story.

Each of us is connected to every Revolutionary Beauty who found the courage to transform her life.

Revolutionary Beauty springs from within, from the age-less, renewable energy streaming through our bodies as we heal ourselves through self-care, healthy whole foods, and positive rituals. Our purpose in writing this book is to free you—not enslave you. This book is **not** about diet and fitness regimens meant to squeeze you into a certain dress size—or any dress for that matter. The protocols we teach alchemize you from the inside out, and what you do with that, we can't wait to hear—and see. We are **never** too old, and it's **never** too late. Think of the word "impossible" as *I'm possible.*

We are solar powered, electrically charged beings of light and water. When we connect as a broadband of pure ener-gy, we are unstoppable. Do you notice that when you focus on something, you begin to see it everywhere? The mind is the most powerful algorithm in the universe. To harness this energy, tune into the highest frequencies of positive mes-saging. Collect a tribe of supportive friends and *detoxifica-tion buddies.* Call them when a junk food goblin attempts to hijack your health regimen or interrupt intermittent fasting.

We wrote this book to revolutionize our state of beauty. Our desire is for you to wake up pain-free and energized. We pre-dict you will glow with self-love and tingle with pride when strangers express shock at your age.

You own your experience of pleasure and receive love again. Imagine how you would feel with the energy of a child. En-vision yourself as a wild, yet wiser version of your boldest self—the teenager who believed anything was possible. Fi-nally, **our legacy** is for **you** to live *an unimaginable life.*

To live an unimaginable life while at war with your body is im-possible. *Talk about aging!* We feel 100 years old when only 55 or 45. Gazing at ageless beauties such as Helen Mirren or Goldie Hawn, we might wonder—*of course she looks beauti-ful! Even if I possessed her infinite resources, would I have the same result?*

When I was 28, I visited the Bragg mentored doctor of my teen years who had cracked the code of my ill-health. Heartbroken to hear that he was suffering from severe, crippling arthritis, I shared my long journey since our last meeting. I expounded on the detoxification protocols that I added to his *prescription* of organic food, as well as regular colonics and lymphatic drainage treatments that flushed two decades of pharmaceutical medications.

Because of this, I metamorphized into a vessel of sustainable health and energy. I also proudly shared with him that I had received my Health Educator's Degree at Hippocrates Health Institute, became certified in colon hydrotherapy, and opened my own practice.

Dr. Pottenger's eyes lit up as we hugged, and he reached for my hands. "Thank you, Julia. But, I don't know if I can do all that. Of course, diet has a lot to do with health. Maybe you healed because you were just meant to be here."

Nearly 40 years and thousands of clients later, I can now tell you that my beloved friend was wrong. I had *good angels* like him, and others, who held a light as I found my way. But my healing was **not** a fluke and is **entirely** duplicatable. My clients have done so. Millions of Bragg followers have done so. And you can heal, as well. I am devoted to sharing this message with anyone and everyone who will listen.

That is my legacy.

What is yours?

Start now. Redefine beauty as how **you** feel about yourself—your *self*, not anyone else. In our culture, for a woman to look in the mirror and smile at her image, is a revolutionary act. Restore your health. Revitalize your beauty. Reinvent your life, one dance move at a time.

Tell your story. Live your dreams. Revolutionary Beauty is **not** skin deep. Genuine beauty penetrates the galaxy like a meteor. This undeniable energy is felt, seen, and experienced—and will live on long after we leave.

Best-selling author and Revolutionary Beauty Marsh Engle writes in her book, *Amazing Woman, Emerge!*

"It's time for a radiant revolution. From how we see things to how we do things, we are transforming our work and our lives. We stand true to our voices, and own the power of creativity as never before, bringing to the fore unique possibilities for contribution and meaning, calling forth our most purpose infused, soul powered, spirit guided lives. The most revolutionary move a woman can make is to put her love into action. The essence of feminine power can and will transform the world."

This is our legacy, our ability to make a mark upon the world, and leave a part of us behind for others to benefit and grow. Earthly matter never disappears, but morphs—ice into water, water seeps into the earth, earth grows a tree. Energy is eternal. Although Vital Force may become dormant, with barely a pulse, it can be revived. *We are the captains of our own ship!* Self-care is healing, which allows us to create ageless renewable energy, unapologetically our own—and that is revolutionary.

To all of you Revolutionary Beauties, we rise together with you!

—Julia Loggins and Patricia Bragg

LIANA WERNER-GRAY

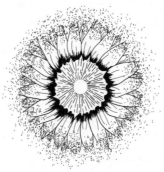

We are excited to share this interview with Liana Werner-Gray, wholistic health expert, nutritionist, and best-selling author of *The Earth Diet*, *Cancer-Free with Food*, and *Anxiety-Free with Food*. Liana healed life-threatening health issues through food.

Julia: Would you share your healing story? It's inspirational!

Liana: *I grew up in the Outback, Alice Springs. Quite natural and healthy. I moved to the city at 18 and started to indulge in a fast-food, junk food lifestyle. The aboriginals taught us the healthiest way to eat was to get food from the trees and the land. I knew from the get-go that junk food was wrong, but food became like a drug. I would get high for five or ten minutes and then crash—it was a vicious cycle. To avoid that bad feeling, I would eat more junk food. It's hard to eat junk food and not binge, right? It makes us want to keep eating and eating, the sugar and fats. Then, I ended up in the hospital at 21 with a golf ball sized tumor in my throat, right in my lymphatic system. It was such a wake-up call. I knew I had to go back to eating natural food and eating food with nutritional value. I did a lot of detoxifiation, juicing, colonics, and coffee enemas.*

Colonics saves lives. It contributed to healing my body, juicing, making my own recipes—chocolate balls—and that's when I came up with The Earth Diet. Every time I had a craving

I thought, how can I make that with natural ingredients? I was healing my body, but fulfilling all the cravings.

I opted out of all conventional treatments. Because of the aboriginals, I knew if you just cut out a tumor and don't address the root cause it will just grow back somewhere else. So, my goal was to heal my body and the source of the tumor. The aboriginals shaped a lot of my career with nature because I grew up with indigenous culture.

I learned the lymph is the body's sewage system and it does such a great job unless we overload it with toxins, and it gets sluggish and creates tumors, and also contributes to breast tumors. A lot of breast cancer comes from toxins in the lymph system. If we eat a diet like The Earth Diet, *we keep our lymph healthy. If we do have a build-up we need to do a detox, colonics, and coffee enemas to clean the gut.*

And, cut out refined sugar. The lymph can't stand it. I healed my body from switching from white sugar. I ate natural sugars to heal my body—replacement therapy. Sugar is a stronger addiction than cocaine; that's been proven. Have some fruit and cut out white sugar. That completely healed my lymphatic system and now, I don't crave sugar the way I used to.

It's easy, everything we want to eat we can use coconut and natural sugar. We want to cut out GMO foods and processed foods in Cancer-Free Foods. *I list the top foods the lymph does not like. Type o people especially need more protein. When they are deficient in protein they crave sugar. When I was living on junk food I didn't have enough protein and the food was ruining my gut. I love hemp seeds. Put them in your smoothies, salads, and soups.*

Julia: Would you tell us about your experience with colonics?

Liana: *It did heal my body. When I tell you about these healing modalities, you will get goosebumps and want to check it out.*

I learned it was done by the Egyptians, and they did it to cleanse and reset the gut. Stuff does accumulate there. It's connected to our brain and immune health. For two months, I did it every other day when I was healing the tumor. But, my gut was so stagnant I wasn't eliminating. I had taken laxatives to move my bowels, so my muscles weren't working. The colon therapist was helping my muscles to work again. It was interesting to see all that stuff that come out, and my friend saw a tumor.

The whole healing process was very emotional. I had to do a lot of healing from my past, and face some traumas from childhood. All of that came up, which was expected. My colon therapist explained to me that it was part of the healing process. I knew I needed to do the physical healing, and I needed to do the emotional healing. What I've learned now is that no matter how hard, dark, and painful it is to heal those traumas, it's worth it all to face these. Not everyone has had trauma, but a lot of people have. It's so healing, and it's a new life when you come out on the other side.

It is a natural cycle, the healing process, and it is a journey. Before I got sick with my tumor, I used to be the kind of person who would say, "Don't talk about negative stuff, don't think about it. Don't feel it." I think that was part of why I got sick—I had to confront that shadow side and heal. I've coached people for 11 years now. I'm a certified nutritionist. If someone has gone through certain traumas—and not all traumas are equal, but everyone goes through some kind of trauma in their life—we have to explore it. And, it can be dark; it's not light. However, it's part of life and the human experience. I've had to do the spiritual warfare myself, and acknowledge that there was darkness, tough experiences I'd had, and not sugarcoat it. I encourage my patients to do the spiritual warfare and acknowledge the darkness and trauma that they went through, or had inflicted upon them.

It's the same with diet. As human beings we do have a right and potential to live in joy every single day, for sure. But, there *are times we do have to deprive ourselves of pleasures in the moment that are't going to lead to healthy, sustainable consequences. There is some suffering, and it's okay to feel that. We can handle it. For example, if we want to eat that chocolate cake and we think, "I'm going to feel amazing for five or ten minutes with dopamine and serotonin," but then, we're gong to suffer after that. And, if not at that moment, we will feel it tomorrow, or years down the road—we will have a health consequence.* **No one** *gets away with eating junk long term. We choose, "I am going to deprive myself now and feel joy later." That's spiritual discipline.*

Julia: How do you support people moving forward rather than retreating on their healing journey?

Liana: *I always tell my patients, use your intuition. If something doesn't sound right, don't do it. I say, make a choice and take a step forward because you'll soon know. God will show you very quickly if it's the right decision. Some people get stuck not making any decision, not moving at all. Not taking any action is worse; it's better to act and learn from it than not. If you have two options, choose one option and take that step. You will very quickly know. God or the Universe will let you know if you should turn back or keep going.*

Julia: What are your personal rituals?

Liana: *The most regular thing I do is I drink a green drink every single day. I implemented that ritual when I was healing. At that time, I was drinking six juices a day when I had the tumor. After three months, the tumor had completely healed. It had completely drained. After that, I said, "Why wouldn't I drink a green juice every single day for the rest of my life? Why not?"*

Green juice has chlorophyll, which under a microscope looks exactly the same as blood cells; except it has magnesium and blood is made of iron. If we want healthy blood we are what we eat. Every time we drink a green juice, our body imprints that; our blood imprints that. The magnesium is so good for relaxing the body and for healing anxiety, depression, and stress. The chlorophyll is packed with oxygen. What does cancer hate the most? Oxygen.

Green juice alkalizes the body. I feel a difference if a day has gone by and I haven't had a green drink yet. If I'm traveling, I mix a green powder with spinach, kale, broccoli, collard greens. I make a fresh juice as much as I can. That one green drink keeps our health consistent forever, and I think every human can commit to that. Think how much healthier we would be if everyone did that.

I do exercise a lot. I had a realization that we have 24 hours in the day so why not spend one hour doing body maintenance. I spend one hour a day doing movement, lifting weights, walking, dancing, something physical—seeing what needs to be worked on, breathing out trapped energy.

Also, I am constantly in conversation with God, and I think that is the biggest part of my practice. As soon as I wake up, I put my spiritual practice at the forefront of my mind and it brings so much joy to my life. I check in with God, with every decision.

I think we each have a gift. Whatever it is, we have to use those gifts. If not, we feel very depressed and we start to slowly die. It makes it fun to get up in the morning. I've been living my purpose for 11 years and I am so grateful. Living your purpose makes you feel like your soul is right where it needs to be. You are doing what you're meant to do. If someone is not learning what their gifts are, say, "I want to live my life where I am utilizing my gifts and my purpose." Set the intention.

You know it because your soul just knows—it's there. I was 28 when I realized I am going to age. I had friends say you're going to work on the inner, and I knew that. Our physical appearance does change. I look forward to the inner peace that comes with each year. I think joy helps us stay youthful longer.

I think society is shifting to embrace health and joy as beautiful. It's all about the inner light. Joy is the most beautiful thing.

Julia: How did you meet Patricia?

Liana: *When I first came to America, ten years ago, it was for my mission of teaching health and wellness. The health industry was bigger here, and I wanted to be part of the revolution. When I first got here, I discovered nutritional yeast, and that became my cheese alternative. I made the kale recipe, and I got into ACV. I saw Patricia on the logo of the package and I thought, wow, this lady is goals. What a legacy! I started going to the food shows. The biggest one was in Anaheim, California. One year I turn around, and there was Patricia. I thought, **no way!** She was tiny, but she looked exactly like she did on the label of her products.*

I said, "I can't believe I'm meeting you in person! Let me tell you about The Earth Diet." We took a photo, and I saw her the next year. Then, I saw Katy Perry, and I made a vegan lasagna with nutritional yeast from Bragg, and we did a video and I felt such a synergy. I was so grateful in March 2020 to make her the superfood kale salad right on her farm. She has such an amazing legacy. She said, "You're the young generation—you have to continue the legacy."

Julia: What does *Revolutionary Beauty* mean to you?

Liana: *I'm so excited about your new book. What it means is, it's a new type of beauty, and when I think of that, I see you—I see Patricia. I think energy, vibrance, and joy. It's energy beauty. It's the energy we're embodying, the joy—**nothing** is more attractive than joy. Just being revolutionary in terms of not getting stuck in an unhealthy version of what beauty is.*

We're in a new era, embracing true health from the inside out. Natural health is not only beauty as far as energy, but for the environment as well. It embraces a clean, healthy environment.

That's revolutionary. The glow comes from what we eat, breathe, what we think, and spirituality is a huge help for that as well. My spiritual relationship is a huge part of my daily life.

I am a huge believer that our pain can drive us to our greatest awakening, as long as we don't run from it. When we turn and face it, and ask for help and say, "God, what am I supposed to learn here?" That is when our lives change. That is when we heal our relationship to our bodies and we love and accept ourselves. And, that is revolutionary!

REVOLUTIONARY BEAUTY RECIPES

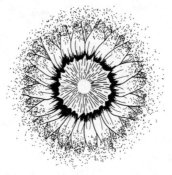

By Liana Werner-Gray

Basic Salad Dressing

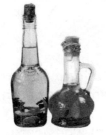

Total time: 5 minutes—makes 1/3 cup

Ingredients
- 1/3 cup oil—extra-virgin olive, coconut, MCT, or avocado
- 2 tbsp. Bragg Apple Cider Vinegar
- 1 tbsp. fresh lemon juice
- Sea salt and pepper

Actions
1. Add all ingredients into a bowl and whisk until well combined. Season with salt and pepper if desired.

Tip
- Refrigerate in airtight container for the dressing to last two months.

Cashew Ice Cream Bites with Chocolate Sauce

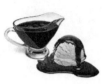

Total time: 10 minutes preparation, plus soaking and freezing—makes 15 bites

Ingredients
- 1 1/2 cups cashews, soak 4 hours
- 1/2 cup maple syrup
- 1 tsp. maca
- 1 tbsp. vanilla extract
- Juice of 1 small lemon (2 to 3 tbsps.)
- Dash of salt
- 1/4 cup refined or extra-virgin coconut oil
- 1 batch of chocolate sauce, as a topping (see chocolate sauce recipe below)

Chocolate Sauce Ingredients
- 2/3 cup cacao powder
- 1/2 cup maple syrup
- 1/4 cup extra-virgin coconut oil

Actions
1. Add cacao, maple syrup, and oil to a blender.
2. Mix on high speed until smooth. Set aside in a bowl.
3. Blend cashew bite ingredients on high until smooth, without lumps.
4. Scoop ice cream mixture into little mounds onto a parchment lined baking tray. Freeze for 5 minutes.
5. Spoon chocolate sauce over ice cream bites. Freeze for 30 minutes and your gourmet dessert is ready!

Tips
- For a smoother creamier ice cream texture be sure to soak the cashews for several hours.
- For a nut-free version, use hempseeds, pumpkin seeds, or sunflower seeds instead of cashews.

Cashew Ice Cream Bites with Chocolate Sauce

- This recipe works well with almonds, macadamia nuts, walnuts, or Brazil nuts.
- You may substitute carob for cocoa.
- You may substitute matcha green tea powder for maca.
- For spice, consider adding a dash of cayenne or cinnamon to chocolate suace.

Cauliflower Popcorn

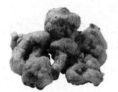

Total time: 10 minutes—serves 4

Ingredients
- 2 1/2 tbsps. extra-virgin olive oil or Nutiva Coconut Oil with Buttery Flavor
- 1/2 cup Bragg nutritional yeast
- 3/4 tsp. sea salt
- 1 head cauliflower, chopped into bite-size pieces

Actions
1. Preheat the oven to 325°F.
2. Mix the oil, nutritional yeast, and salt in a large bowl until combined. Place cauliflower into the mixture and toss until pieces are well coated.
3. Place cauliflower onto a baking tray and bake for 20 minutes, or until golden brown.

Tips
- For extra flavor, add 1 tablespoon sesame seeds.
- For extra protein, add 1 tablespoon SunButter.
- Use Nutiva Coconut Oil with Buttery Flavor for a *movie popcorn* flavor.

Thai Chicken Pizza

Total time: 1 hour—serves 4

Ingredients
- 1/3 cup organic SunButter
- 3 tbsp. filtered water
- 1 tbsp. Bragg Liquid Aminos
- 1 tbsp. lime juice
- 1 tbsp. honey
- 1 garlic clove, crushed
- 1 tsp. minced ginger
- Red pepper flakes, to taste (optional)
- 1 tbsp. coconut oil, for frying
- 1 large organic chicken breast, diced
- 1 prepared pizza crust (organic or gluten-free crust)
- 1 cup organic or vegan mozzarella cheese
- 3 scallions, chopped

Actions
1. Preheat oven to 450°F.
2. In a saucepan, combine SunButter, water, liquid aminos, lime juice, honey, garlic, ginger, and red pepper flakes. Cook over medium. Stir until well combined.
3. Add oil and chicken to frying pan. When the chicken turns white, pour half the sauce over chicken. Cook until chicken is done through the middle.
4. Place the pizza crust on a full sheet pan. Spread remaining sauce over crust. Cover crust with 3/4 cup cheese, then add chicken and scallions. Sprinkle remaining 1/4 cup cheese on top of the pizza.
5. Bake pizza for 12-15 minutes until cheese is melted and crust is fully cooked and crisp.
6. Garnish with fresh cilantro and red pepper flakes.

Tip
- Grain-free pizza crusts work well, too!

Cashew Cheese

Total time: 10 minutes—serves 1 (1/4 cup each)

Ingredients
- 2 cups cashews
- 2 tbsp. Bragg Nutritional Yeast
- 1/2 tsp. sea salt
- Juice of 1 small lemon (no more than 1/4 cup)
- 1/2 cup filtered water (more for a softer cheese)

Actions
1. Blend all ingredients in a food processor until mixture is smooth. Add more water if a softer cheese is desired.

Tips
- Soak cashews for 4 hours for a smoother, creamier cheese.
- For a nut-free version, use hempseeds, pumpkin seeds, or sunflower seeds instead of cashews.
- This recipe also works well with almonds, macadamia nuts, walnuts, or Brazil nuts.
- For a cheesier flavor, add more nutritional yeast. You can also make this recipe without nutritional yeast.
- Add a dash of cayenne or chili flakes for spice.
- Add 1 teaspoon thyme for more flavor.

Variations
- To make raw Parmesan cheese, add additional 3 tablespoons nutritional yeast to mixture and spread to 1/4-inch thick on a dehydrator tray. Place in a food dehydrator for 12 hours. It will crumble easily when you are ready to use it.
- Add 1 garlic clove or more for Garlic Cashew Cheese.
- Add 1 cup fresh basil leaves for Pesto Cashew Cheese.

Creamy Vegan Gluten-Free Mac n' Cheese

Total time: 20 minutes—serves 4

Ingredients
- 2 garlic cloves
- 1/4 cup tapioca starch flour
- 1/2 tsp. sea salt
- 1/4 tsp. thyme
- 1/4 tsp. rosemary
- 1/4 tsp. black pepper
- 2 cups almond milk or other nut milk
- 1/4 cup Bragg Nutritional Yeast
- 1 box Explore Cuisine Chickpea Fusilli
- 3 tbsps. raw Parmesan cheese or store-bought vegan Parmesan (optional)
- 1/4 cup Nutiva Coconut Oil with Buttery Flavor

Actions
1. Cook pasta per directions. Drain and set aside.
2. While pasta is cooking, heat oil over medium heat in a medium cooking pot. Add garlic, and cook for 2 minutes until golden. Add in arrowroot tapioca flour starch and whisk for 1 minute. Slowly add in almond milk while whisking. Continue to cook over medium heat for 2 minutes.
3. Whisk in nutritional yeast and vegan Parmesan, if using. Sauce will be a little clumpy at first, so keep stirring in milk until completely smooth. You can also use a hand blender or transfer mixture into a blender if you want a smoother consistency.
4. Add pasta to pot of hot sauce and mix well with the seasonings. Then, serve in bowls.

Creamy Vegan Gluten-Free Mac n' Cheese

Tips
- Serve with toppings you like. I love adding organic peas, corn, chopped fresh parsley, and dried chili pepper to mine.
- If you intend to use raw Parmesan cheese, then make sure to prepare a day ahead since it takes 12 hours to make in a dehydrator. Store-bought is a convenience.

Superfood Kale Salad

Total time: 10 minutes—serves 3

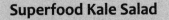

Ingredients
- 1 peeled avocado
- 1 tbsp. Bragg Apple Cider Vinegar
- 2 tsps. Bragg Liquid Aminos
- 1 1/2 tsps. Nutiva MCT or flaxseed oil
- 4 tbsp. Bragg Nutritional Yeast
- 2 tbsp. SunButter sunflower seed butter
- 1 bunch of kale, center ribs, and stems removed

Actions
1. In a large bowl, tear kale leaves into small pieces.
2. Massage the avocado into pieces of kale with your fingers, covering the kale with avocado.
3. Add remaining ingredients to bowl and stir. Or, continue massaging mixture until well combined.

Tip
- For sensitive tummies, lightly steam the kale

Blueberry Muffins

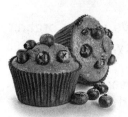

Total time: 50 minutes—serves 12

Ingredients
- 2 tbsps. flax meal
- 2 tbsps. filtered water
- 1/2 cup almond milk
- 1/3 cup maple syrup
- 1 tsp. Bragg Apple Cider Vinegar
- 1 1/2 tsps. baking soda
- 2 organic apples or 1/2 cup unsweetened applesauce
- 1 tbsp. MCT oil
- 1/4 cup coconut oil
- 1/4 cup coconut sugar
- 1/2 tsp. sea salt
- 1 cup organic blueberries
- 2 tbsps. chia seeds

Gluten-Free Flour Mix Ingredients
- 1 tbsp. potato starch
- 2 tbsps. tapioca starchflour
- 1/4 cup tigernut flour
- 1 tbsp. brown rice flour
- 3/4 cup Nutiva plant based protein powder
- 1/4 cup almond flour

Actions
1. Preheat oven to 375°F and line a 12-cup muffin tray with paper baking cups.
2. Make an egg replacement: Mix flax and water together in a small cup until well combined. Let mixture sit for 10 minutes until it becomes gummy like an egg. Set aside.
3. Combine all ingredients of gluten-free flour mix in a separate bowl and set aside.

Blueberry Muffins

4. Mix the almond milk, apple cider vinegar, and baking soda in a separate bowl until well combined. Set aside.
5. Peel and core apples. Mix in a blender or food processor with MCT oil until you create applesauce.
6. Mix coconut oil, maple syrup, coconut sugar, and applesauce in a separate large bowl. Add egg replacement (see step 2) to mixture and whisk.
7. Add almond milk mixture and stir well.
8. Add sea salt, gluten-free flour mix, and stir well.
9. Gently stir in blueberries and chia seeds.
10. Pour batter evenly among 12 baking cups and bake for 24 minutes, or until golden brown. Insert a toothpick into the center of a muffin to test. If toothpick is dry, then the muffins are cooked.
11. Let muffins cool for 15 minutes and enjoy!

Tips
- For nut-allergies, use rice milk instead of almond milk.
- If you prefer a banana flavor, substitute 2 mashed bananas for applesauce.
- To achieve a zero glycemic content, substitute 1/4 cup monk fruit powder for the coconut sugar.
- Substitute coconut flour for tiger nut flour

Chocolate Hazelnut Cake

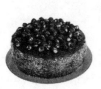

Total time: 1 hour and 10 minutes—serves 16

Cake Ingredients
- 1 tbsp. baking soda
- 1 tsp. Bragg Apple Cider Vinegar
- 1/4 cup flaxseed meal
- 3 apples, peeled and cored
- 1/2 cup plus 2 tbsps. filtered water
- 2/3 cup coconut sugar
- 1/2 cup plus 2 tbsps. maple syrup
- 1 tsp. vanilla extract
- 1/2 tsp. salt
- 1/2 cup coconut oil, refined or extra-virgin
- 1 cup cacao powder
- 1 1/2 cups almond flour
- 1 cup oat flour (or blended oats to a fine flour)
- 1/2 cup tapioca flour
- 1 cup almond milk or another plant based milk (use seed milk in case of nut allergy)

Frosting Ingredients
- 1 1/2 cups organic powdered sugar
- 1/2 cup almond milk
- 1/2 cup cacao powder
- 1/4 cup maple syrup
- 1/4 cup Nutiva Coconut Oil with Buttery Flavor or extra-virgin coconut oil

Topping Ingredients
- 1 cup roasted hazelnuts, chopped
- 1/2 cup roasted walnuts, chopped

Chocolate Hazelnut Cake

Actions

1. Preheat oven to 350°F, and grease a round cake pan.
2. Add almond milk, baking soda, and apple cider vinegar to a large bowl. Stir and let mixture sit a few minutes to curdle.
3. Add flax meal and water to a separate bowl. Whisk together well, then set aside.
4. In 5 minutes, the texture will be gummy like eggs.
5. Blend apples in a food processor until you have applesauce.
6. Add flax meal mixture, applesauce, coconut sugar, and maple syrup to almond milk bowl. Whisk.
7. Add vanilla, salt, and coconut oil, then stir.
8. Add almond flour, oat flour, and tapioca flour. Whisk together.
9. Whisk together the cacao powder and flours in a separate bowl. Add to wet mixture, stir gently.
10. Pour batter into cake pan. Bake for 40 to 45 minutes. Let cool in the tin before removing from pan.
11. Make frosting in a bowl or blender by whipping together all ingredients until thick and smooth. When cake is completely cooled, smooth the frosting onto the cake.
12. Garnish outside of cake with hazelnuts and walnuts. Enjoy!

Tips

- If allergic to apples, use two mashed bananas
- 1/2 cup monk fruit powder can be substituted for maple syrup
- Walnut oil may be exchanged for coconut oil
- Powdered sugar comes in sugar-free varieties

Bean Burgers

Total time: 20 minutes—serves 4

Ingredients
- 1 small yellow onion, chopped
- 1 tbsp. Bragg Nutritional Yeast
- 2 tbsps. broccoli sprouts, diced
- 1 tsp. black seeds
- 1/2 tsp. cumin
- 1/4 tsp. garlic powder
- 1/4 tsp. fennel
- 1/4 tsp. thyme
- 1/4 tsp. sage
- 1/4 tsp. sea salt
- 1/4 tsp. black pepper
- 1/8 tsp. turmeric
- Pinch of cayenne pepper
- 1 Flax Egg Alternative
- 2 tbsps. extra-virgin coconut oil
- 1/2 cup almond meal (blended almond)
- 1 x 15-ounce can organic beans (butter or black beans)

Actions
1. Drain beans. Mash beans in a bowl and mix in remaining ingredients, except for oil. Taste mixture and add spices or sea salt to your liking. Divide mixture and shape into 4 patties.
2. Heat oil in large pan over medium heat. Fry patties until golden—about 5 minutes on each side.
3. Serve on gluten-free tortillas, kale, collard greens, or lettuce. Burgers taste great with herbs such as fresh parsley, cilantro, and basil.

Tips
- Non vegans can use 1 egg instead of Flax Egg.
- Replace almond meal with pumpkin seed meal.

Grass-Fed Beef Burritos

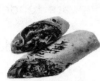

Total time: 25 minutes—serves 6 (1 burrito each)

Ingredients
- 2 tbsps. extra-virgin olive oil
- 1/2 tsp. turmeric powder
- 1/4 tsp. black pepper
- 1 pound ground grass fed beef
- 1 small yellow onion, chopped
- 2 large garlic cloves, diced
- 1 1/2 tsps. ground cumin
- 1/2 tsp. turmeric powder
- 1/4 tsp. sea salt
- 1/4 tsp. pepper
- 1 tsp. chili powder or cayenne pepper
- 6 brown rice tortillas or wraps

Filling Ingredients
- 3/4 cup Vegan Sour Cream
- 1 cup Bragg Nutritional Yeast
- 1/2 cup grated carrot
- Diced lettuce
- 1 avocado, cubed
- 1 pepper, diced
- Fresh cilantro, chopped Broccoli sprouts
- 16 ounces black beans (soaked, cooked, soft)

Actions
1. Heat a large frying pan with oil over medium heat. Add turmeric and black pepper. Sauté for 1 minute or until sizzling. Add beef and cook for 3 to 4 minutes or until brown. Stir frequently.
2. Add onion, garlic, cumin, turmeric powder, sea salt, pepper, and chili powder to meat. Stir.

Grass-Fed Beef Burritos

3. Cook for 7 minutes or until vegetables are tender and flavors are well combined.
4. Place 1/4 cup of meat into each tortilla and then add your fillings of choice.

Tips
- If you want to take it a step further, heat the oven to 375°F, fully assemble your burrito and then place on parchment paper and bake for 12 minutes, until burritos have turned golden brown.
- Add 1/4 cup raw tomato sauce to beef.

Variations
- Use chicken for chicken burritos.
- Use fish for fish burritos.
- Use beans and vegetable stir-fry for veggie burritos.

ABOUT JULIA LOGGINS

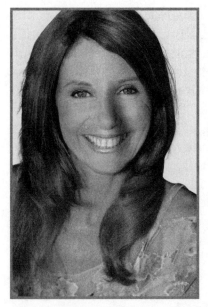

Digestive Health Expert Julia Loggins began the study of holistic health when inspired by saving her own life after a childhood of life-threatening illnesses. In 1983, she received her Health Educator's Certification, and studied the mind-body connection with Dr. Ernest Pecci, whose work continues at the Hoffman Institute.

Founded by Ms. Loggins 35 years ago, her private practice attracts clients whose health depends on detoxification and regenerative nutrition. She holds international certifications in colon hydrotherapy, regenerative nutrition, and fertility health.

The Unimaginable Life, written with former husband Kenny Loggins launched her writing career. As her practice grew, she wrote *Dare to Detoxify*, followed a few years later by a practical workbook entitled, *It Takes Guts to be Happy A 21-Day Cleansing Plan to Heal Your Belly & Recharge Your Life.*

In 2017, Julia designed a line of of digestive health and nutritional supplements for sensitive people. She also launched two online courses with live weekly Zoom calls—The Happy Gut Makeover and The Menopause Makeover. She is dedicated to the message of health, happiness, and the leap of transforming the culture of beauty through her books, courses, and consultations.

Mother of two grown children, Julia lives in Santa Barbara with her husband, Paul Turner.

ABOUT PATRICIA BRAGG

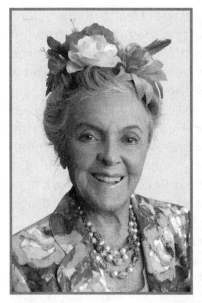

A maverick with a mission, Patricia Bragg's simple, authentic message of health and happiness through natural living has inspired generations, saved lives and influenced the thinking of health care practitioners worldwide. She ran Bragg Live Foods, her pioneering natural foods company, for 65 years and built a health food store condiment into a multimillion-dollar company.

A dedicated health crusader with a passion like her father, Paul C. Bragg, a world-renowned health authority. Patricia achieved international fame in her own right. She spread the word of health worldwide through lectures, radio shows, and magazine interviews throughout her career. She and her father coauthored the Bragg 8-book Health Library of instructive, inspiring books, including the best seller, *Miracle of Fasting*, known as the faster's bible. Patricia lives on a thriving organic farm in Santa Barbara, California.

Other Books by Julia Loggins

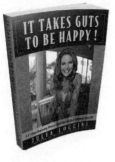 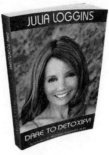 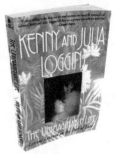

Other Books by
Paul Bragg & Patricia Bragg

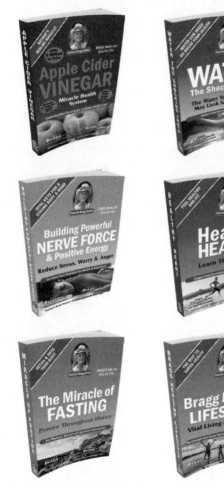 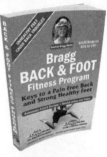 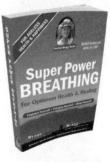 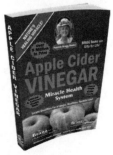

RESOURCE GUIDE

MODULE 1—MINDSET

Revolutionary Beauty—Lisa Proctor-Hawkins
WEBSITE: firefly180.com

Revolutionary Beauty—Marsh Engle
WEBSITE: marshengle.com | theamazingwomannation.com
INSTAGRAM: @marshengle | | @amazingwomannation

Revolutionary Beauty—Tracey Magill
EMAIL: magill.tracey@gmail.com

Dr. Nicole LePera
WEBSITE: linktr.ee/the.holistic.psychologist
BOOK: *How to Do the Work*
INSTAGRAM: @the.holistic.psychologist

Emotional Freedom Technique (EFT)—emofree.com

Eye Movement Desensitization and Reprogramming (EMDR)
WEBSITE: emdr.com

Foundation for Peripheral Neuropathy—foundationforpn.org

Headspace—headspace.com

HeartMath—heartmath.com

Healing Tree—healingtree.com

Hoffman Institute—hoffmaninstitute.org

Moriah Norris-Hale
WEBSITE: theskyinside.net/work-with-me

Joe Dispenza
WEBSITE: drjoedispenza.com

Luke Storey—The Lifestyle Podcast
WEBSITE: lukestorey.com/lifestylistpodcast

MODULE 2—PURIFY

Revolutionary Beauty—Alyson Charles
WEBSITE: alysoncharles.com
INSTAGRAM: @iamalysoncharles

Revolutionary Beauty—Cynthia James
WEBSITE: cynthiajames.net
INSTAGRAM: @cynthiajames777

Revolutionary Beauty—Julia Loggins
    WEBSITE: daretodetoxify.com
    BOOK: *It Takes Guts to be Happy!*
    BOOK: *Dare to Detoxify!*
    DIY RESOURCES FROM JULIA:
        Home Enema: daretodetoxify.com/home-enema
        Coffee Enema: daretodetoxify.com/coffee-enema
        21 Days of Free Happy Gut Tips:
        daretodetoxify.com/21-days-happy-gut-tips
    QUIZZES:
        Parasites Quiz: daretodetoxify.com/parasite-quiz
        Happy Gut Quiz: daretodetoxify.com/happy-gut-quiz
    COURSES:
        Happy Gut Makeover:
        cleansingforenergy.com/pages/happy-gut-makeover
        Mastering Menopause Makeover:
        cleansingforenergy.com/pages/mastering-menopause
    HERBAL FORMULAS:
        Happy Gut Cleanse—Colon and liver cleanse
        Yeast Be Gone—Candida support

Zach Bush, MD
    WEBSITE: linktr.ee/zachbushmd

HerScan Breast Ultrasound
    WEBSITE: herscan.com

Michael Galitzer, MD
    WEBSITE: drgalitzer.com

Gentle Wellness Center—gentlewellnesscenter.com

Gerson Institute—gerson.org/gerpress

I-ACT National Colon Therapy Network—i-act.org

Lisa Levitt Gainsley, CLT
    BOOK: *The Book of Lymph*

Lymphatic Therapy Santa Barbara
    WEBSITE: lymphatictherapysantabarbara.com
    INSTAGRAM: @lymphatictherapysantabarbara

The Nap Ministry
    WEBSITE: linktr.ee/thenapministry

Naturally Recovering Autism
    WEBSITE: naturallyrecoveringautism.com

Perry Nickelston
    WEBSITE: https://www.stopchasingpain.com/
    INSTAGRAM: @stopchasingpain

France Robert, Colon Health
WEBSITE: wellnessbyfrancerobert.com

Elisa Song, MD
WEBSITE: healthykidshappykids.com

Wim Hof Method—wimhofmethod.com

MODULE 3—FASTING

Hippocrates Health Institute—hippocratesinst.org

We Care Spa—wecarespa.com

Sanoviv Medical Institute—sanoviv.com

MODULE 4—FUELING

Revolutionary Beauty—Kelly LeBrock
INSTAGRAM: @thekellylebrock

Revolutionary Beauty—Caroline MacDougall—Teeccino
WEBSITE: teeccino.com
INSTAGRAM: @teeccino

Revolutionary Beauty—Liana Werner-Gray
WEBSITE: linktr.ee/lianawernergray
BOOK: *The Earth Diet*
INSTAGRAM: @lianawernergray

Emily Daniels
WEBSITE: linktr.ee/wholesomehedonista

Mark Hyman, MD
WEBSITE: drmarkhyman.com
BOOK: *The Pegan Diet*

Nisha Melvani
WEBSITE: linktr.ee/cookingforpeanuts
INSTAGRAM: @cookingforpeanuts

MODULE 5—FITNESS

Revolutionary Beauty—Cheri Clampett, C-IAYT
WEBSITE: therapeuticyoga.com/cheri-clampett
INSTAGRAM: @therapeuticyogatraining

Revolutionary Beauty—Elaine LaLanne
WEBSITE: elainelalanne.com

Revolutionary Beauty—Josette Tkacik
WEBSITE: josettetkacik.com
INSTAGRAM: @josettetkacik

Box Union—boxunion.com

CorePower Yoga—corepoweryoga.com

Model Mugging—modelmugging.org

Openfit Pilates—openfit.com

Santa Barbara Beach Yoga
WEBSITE: linktr.ee/santabarbarabeachyoga
INSTAGRAM: @santabarbarabeachyoga

MODULE 6—HORMONES AND SENSUALITY

Revolutionary Beauty—Dr. Leigh Connealy, MD
WEBSITE: connealymd.com
INSTAGRAM: @connealymd

Revolutionary Beauty—Dr. Kathlyn Hendricks
WEBSITE: hendricks.com/about/our-story

Flo Living
WEBSITE: floliving.com

Christine Northrup
WEBSITE: drnorthrup.com

Sara Reardon, PT
WEBSITE: linktree/thevaginawhisperer

Sex with Emily
WEBSITE: sexwithemily.com
INSTAGRAM: @sexwithemily

MODULE 7—SKINCARE AND BEAUTY

Revolutionary Beauty—Erin Elizabeth
WEBSITE: healthnutnews.com

Revolutionary Beauty—Erin Foster
WEBSITE: shopfavoritedaughter.com
INSTAGRAM: @erinfoster

Revolutionary Beauty—Dr. Julia T. Hunter, MD
WEBSITE: juliathuntermd.com
INSTAGRAM: @wholisticdermatology

Revolutionary Beauty—Malea Rose—Vie En Rose
WEBSITE: vieenrose.com
INSTAGRAM: @vieenrosebeauty

True Botanicals—https://truebotanicals.com/

Nourish Organic—https://nourishorganic.com/

OSEA—oseamalibu.com

COOKBOOKS

Half Baked Harvest Cookbook by Tieghan Gerard

The Autoimmune Protocol Comfort Food Cookbook by Michelle Hoover
The Well Plated Cookbook by Erin Clarkel

The Wildly Affordable Organic Cookbook by Linda Watson

ENERGY MEDICINE

International Society for the Study of Subtle Energies and Energy (ISSEEM)—issseem.org | issseemblog.org

Occidental Institute Research Foundation (OIRF)—oirf.com

Physica Energetics—physicaenergetics.com

Root Cause Clinic—rootcauseclinic.co

ENVIRONMENTAL MEDICINE

Academy of Comprehensive Integrative Medicine (ACIM)
WEBSITE: acimconnect.com

American Academy of Environmental Medicine (AAEM)
WEBSITE: aaemonline.org

Gust Environmental—gustenviro.com

HOMEOPATHY

The American Institute of Homeopathy—homeopathyusa.org

National Center for Homeopathy—homeopathycenter.org

PROFESSIONAL RESOURCES—ORGANIZATIONS

American Academy of Anti Aging Medicine (A4M)—A4M.com

American College for Advancement in Medicine (ACAM)
WEBSITE: acam.org

American Academy of Medical Acupuncture (AAMA)
WEBSITE: medicalacupuncture.org

American Board of Integrative Holistic Medicine (ABIHM)
WEBSITE: abihm.org | holisticboard.org

American Holistic Medical Association (AHMA)
WEBSITE: holisticmedicine.org

International College of Applied Kinesiology (ICAK)
WEBSITE: icakusa.com | icak.com

PROFESSIONAL RESOURCES—DENTISTS

International Academy of Biological Dentistry and Medicine (IABDM)—iabdm.org

PROFESSIONAL RESOURCES—PUBLISHING

Deborah S. Nelson—Writing and Publishing Coach
WEBSITE: deborahsnelson.com | publishingSOLO.com
INSTAGRAM: @deborahsnelon

IMAGE CREDITS

Macaroni and Cheese—Matthew Antonino
Cream Cheese—Tobi
Bean Burrito—Maksim Shebeko
Veggie Burger—Nina Firsova
Blueberry Muffins—Mykola Davydenko
Pizza—Boris Ryzhkov
Salad Dressing—Viktoriia Borysenko
Ice Cream with Chocolate Sauce—Unal Ozmen
Fried Cauliflower—Paul Cowan
Kale Salad—Brian Zanchi
Hazelnut Cake—Irina Kryvasheina
Food Combining Chart—DS Publishing
Lymphatic System—Peter Lamb
Colon Diagram—masia8